Introduction to Cognitive Ethnography and Systematic Field Work

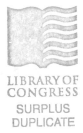

Dr. Cristina Karmas, Professor of English, Graceland University

The wisdom and experience evidenced in statements emphasize, for example, flexibility and serendipity, which must reassure even the most diffident student—who must develop the skills/abilities needed to "plan for the unplanned," to expect the unexpected.

Landon Hancock, Kent State University

It provides an interesting review and cookbook for an apparently underutilized interviewing and analysis method.

Anthony Kwame, Harrison College

Having a road map to transcribing, decision modeling, and creating taxonomic trees is invaluable. In my view, the other sections of the book either build up to or build off of this key centerpiece.

David A. Kinney, Central Michigan University

The author aptly and consistently emphaszes the importance of "controlling researcher bias" and systematically addressing ethical issues throughout the proposal, which is particularly important given the current climate surrounding research.

Sara Miller McCune founded SAGE Publishing in 1965 to support the dissemination of usable knowledge and educate a global community. SAGE publishes more than 1000 journals and over 800 new books each year, spanning a wide range of subject areas. Our growing selection of library products includes archives, data, case studies and video. SAGE remains majority owned by our founder and after her lifetime will become owned by a charitable trust that secures the company's continued independence.

Los Angeles | London | New Delhi | Singapore | Washington DC | Melbourne

Introduction to Cognitive Ethnography and Systematic Field Work

G. Mark Schoepfle

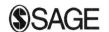

Los Angeles | London | New Delhi
Singapore | Washington DC | Melbourne

QUALITATIVE RESEARCH METHODS SERIES

Series Editor: David L. Morgan, *Portland State University*

The *Qualitative Research Methods Series* currently consists of 60 volumes that address essential aspects of using qualitative methods across the social and behavioral sciences. These widely used books provide valuable resources for a broad range of scholars, researchers, teachers, students, and community-based researchers.

The Series publishes volumes that

- address topics of current interest to the field of qualitative research;

- provide practical guidance and assistance with collecting and analyzing qualitative data;

- highlight essential issues in qualitative research, including strategies to address those issues; and

- add new voices to the field of qualitative research.

A key characteristic of the Qualitative Research Methods Series is an emphasis on both a *"why to"* and a *"how-to"* perspective, so that readers will understand the purposes and motivations behind a method, as well as the practical and technical aspects of using that method. These relatively short and inexpensive books rely on a cross-disciplinary approach, and they typically include examples from practice; tables, boxes, and figures; discussion questions; application activities; and further reading sources.

New and forthcoming volumes in the Series:

Qualitative Instrument Design: A Guide for the Novice Researcher
Felice D. Billups

How to Write a Phenomenological Dissertation
Katarzyna Peoples

Reflexive Narrative: Self-Inquiry Towards Self-Realization and Its Performance
Christopher Johns

Hybrid Ethnography: Online, Offline, and In Between
Liz Przybylski

Thinking and Writing About Qualitative Research

For information on how to submit a proposal for the Series, please contact

- David L. Morgan, Series Editor: morgand@pdx.edu

- Leah Fargotstein, Acquisitions Editor, SAGE: leah.fargotstein@ sagepub.com

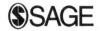

FOR INFORMATION:

SAGE Publications, Inc.
2455 Teller Road
Thousand Oaks, California 91320
E-mail: order@sagepub.com

SAGE Publications Ltd.
1 Oliver's Yard
55 City Road
London, EC1Y 1SP
United Kingdom

SAGE Publications India Pvt. Ltd.
B 1/I 1 Mohan Cooperative Industrial Area
Mathura Road, New Delhi 110 044
India

SAGE Publications Asia-Pacific Pte. Ltd.
18 Cross Street #10-10/11/12
China Square Central
Singapore 048423

Printed in the United States of America

Library of Congress Cataloging-in-Publication Data

Names: Schoepfle, G. Mark, author.

Title: Introduction to cognitive ethnography and systematic field work / G. Mark Schoepfle.

Description: Los Angeles : Sage, 2022. | Series: Qualitative research methods series | Includes bibliographical references and index.

Identifiers: LCCN 2021002578 | ISBN 9781544351018 (paperback) | ISBN 9781544351032 (epub) | ISBN 9781544351049 (epub) | ISBN 9781544351025 (ebook)

Subjects: LCSH: Interviewing in ethnology. | Anthropological linguistics. | Ethnology—Fieldwork—Methodology.

Classification: LCC GN346.3 .S35 2022 | DDC 305.8—dc23

LC record available at https://lccn.loc.gov/2021002578

This book is printed on acid-free paper.

Sponsoring Editor: Leah Fargotstein
Product Associate: Kenzie Offley
Production Editor: Natasha Tiwari; Astha Jaiswal
Copy Editor: QuADS Prepress Pvt. Ltd.
Typesetter: Hurix Digital
Proofreader: Theresa Kay
Indexer: Integra
Cover Designer: Janet Kiesel
Marketing Manager: Victoria Velasquez

MIX
Paper from responsible sources
FSC
www.fsc.org
FSC® C008955

21 22 23 24 25 10 9 8 7 6 5 4 3 2 1

BRIEF CONTENTS

DETAILED CONTENTS

PREFACE

This book provides instruction for conducting cognitive ethnography and analyzing the data that are gathered from it. The strength of this approach is the theoretical base that allows interviews to be both flexible and systematic. They are flexible because they are designed to be structured around the semantic knowledge being elicited from the speaker, not around some preconceived design that is based on the researcher's background. They are rigorous because the basic linguistic and semantic structures are shared among all cultures. Thus, accountability is both possible and required. An additional benefit of this cognitive ethnographic method is that interview and classroom instruction can be closely coordinated through teaching and praxis.

Although this book leans heavily on ethnographic examples from studies of the Navajo culture, it also stresses that this method can be applied to one's own culture, with great improvements in the results. Regardless of the culture, the people being interviewed are consultants, not subjects, because they are the experts on the knowledge being obtained from them.

This book is divided into eight chapters. An examination of these chapters reflects that both instruction and demonstration of interviews and analysis are closely intertwined. Chapter 1 orients the reader to a basic definition of ethnography in general and cognitive ethnography in particular. Notably, it stresses that the primary goal is the description of another people's knowledge from the standpoint of their language, even when the language of the people being studied is the same as the researcher's. Thus, students of cognitive ethnography can quickly put their classroom instruction to use. It also disciplines the reader to separate the notes of their observation from those obtained from interview. Both are important but need to be kept separate.

Chapter 2 discusses the planning of a research project. While ethnographic research is fraught with uncertainty, it is still necessary to plan carefully about the types of equipment to be taken, who will conduct the research, what the ethnographers would like to learn, with whom the ethnographers will conduct their inquiry, where the research will be conducted, how long it might take, and when would be the most feasible time to conduct it. This chapter also discusses the number of people to interview, how to select or sample them, and how to treat native research colleagues and interpreters. Finally, it outlines how to compose research teams and how to integrate those being studied with the research design.

Chapter 3 provides an orientation to the semantic unity of *modification*, *taxonomy*, and *queuing* (MTQ). These semantic relationships are at the center of both eliciting and analyzing interview data. This chapter thus demonstrate how to conduct and analyze ethnographic interviews through schematic diagrams centered on the MTQ schema.

Chapter 4 concentrates on the natural history of the ethnographic interview itself. It describes how ethnographers can structure an interview iteratively around the knowledge described by a consultant. It also describes how ethnographers can ask questions that ascertain this knowledge and build interviews around it. Thus, an interview is systematic and structured, with the structure being built around the knowledge of the consultant. As a result, this book stresses that analysis and interview elicitation follow closely, one upon the other.

Chapter 5 builds on Chapters 3 and 4 and shows how to combine these basic semantic relationships into more complex semantic models such as cause–effect, part–whole, and implication. It also shows how to combine taxonomy and queuing when studying decision making and applying decision modeling.

Chapter 6 digresses to some of the basics on how to transcribe interviews and journals. It also outlines how to monitor good translations. The section shows in practical terms how to accurately transcribe not only the ethnographer's personal field notes, or journal, but also the recorded interviews. The chapter concludes with an example of the intricacies of translation. While not a detailed instruction on how to translate, the chapter illustrates how translation proceeds. It also shows how translation can follow into ethnographic analysis and specifies the reasons why translation should never be taken for granted.

Chapter 7 touches briefly on observation. Observation is the first activity an ethnographer conducts when working among any new group of people. This chapter acknowledges that it is not possible to understand a body of cultural knowledge from interview alone any more than it is by observation alone. Nevertheless, it will show that uninformed observations, no matter how systematic, set more traps through bias and distortion than interviews. This chapter also emphasizes the need for keeping observation journals separate from interview transcriptions. It concludes by discussing how the interplay between interview and observation gives rise to what anthropologists call participant observation. It shows that when both interview and observation are monitored carefully the result can be very informative. Additionally, Chapter 7 throws into sharp relief the need for factual accuracy. The researcher should promote, as far as possible, the same standards from consultants as eyewitnesses as from their own observations.

Chapter 8 discusses how to apply the ethnographic process to facilitate writing a final report. The actual form of the written report may be fixed by the institution that supported or requested the ethnography. Nevertheless, it can be made easier by using the description generated from the MTQ schema as a point of departure. The coresearchers may also assume responsibility for giving presentations to both academic and local audiences.

BACKGROUND

This book follows from the 1987 book *Systematic Fieldwork* by Oswald Werner, Mark Schoepfle, and others. It is an outgrowth of a 1974 research project on Navajo student life in the Reservation schools, operated by what was then the Navajo Tribe's Division of Education, then under the direction of Dillon Platero.

Although this project was funded by the National Institute of Education, it was under the control and management of the Navajo Tribe. Werner and I hired and trained Navajos as ethnographers to gather and analyze the data and to jointly write the reports. Other Navajo researchers who had worked with Werner on earlier projects further trained the new staff in transcription and analysis. They also trained me in Navajo transcription and assisted in developing the research strategy and technique.

During the 1970s and early 1980s, I migrated this cognitive ethnographic approach, through similar federally funded research, to what was then Navajo Community College, Shiprock Campus (today Diné College). The projects were funded through contracts and grants with the Environmental Protection Agency, National Science Foundation, National Institutes of Health, and National Institute of Education. All of these were operated by Navajo-controlled institutions. The college motivated Navajo students to present their research to regional academic organizations such as the American Association for the Advancement of Science, the Western Social Sciences Association, and the American Anthropological Association.

These projects benefited from the Navajos who were trained under the previous projects. These researchers thus took on greater importance and influence for researcher training; data analysis, interpretation, and presentation; and project direction. Chief among them were Martha Austin-Garrison, Kenneth Begishe, Frank Morgan, Rose Morgan, and Kenneth Nabahe. Others included Johnny John, Henry Thomas, Beverly Tso, Kee Yazzie, Laura Roan, Angela Johnson, Lucie Upshaw, William Collins, Rita Oquita, Isabelle Zohnnie, David Salt, and Jennifer King. The college also participated actively in the Northwestern University Field School of Ethnography. In addition to enlisting Navajo students, this program also placed non-Navajo college students in various tribal and federal government institutions throughout the Navajo Nation.

This book also needs to acknowledge the contributions of Edward Garrison, Mark Bauer, James McNeley, Philip Reno, Martin Topper, and Shiprock Campus director James Tutt during the Diné College research. Special mention also needs to be made of Michael Burton, without whom the symbiosis between cognitive ethnographic and statistical approaches would not have been actuated, even though this connection had long been recognized as possible.

This brief history especially needs to acknowledge the mentorship of Professor Oswald Werner. Through his vision and diplomatic skills, he proposed and obtained federal funding for the *Six Navajo School Ethnographies* (Werner et al., 1976) and continued his pioneering work through research in other cultures. He also ensured that Navajo tribal and educational control of research projects resulted in research of the highest quality. Without his critique and advice, neither would this book have been written, nor would the resources from the two-volume *Systematic Fieldwork* (Werner & Schoepfle, 1987a, 1987b) have been readily available.

I also extend gratitude to Jennifer Talken-Spaulding, National Park Service Bureau cultural anthropologist, Cultural Anthropology Program, for the release of interview transcripts for use in this volume. Also, thanks is due to Scott Gustafson and Philip Herr, who reviewed this book. Special mention also needs to be made of Elizabeth Schoepfle for her tireless work in clarifying this book's basic writing and for having the nerve both to criticize the writing and to propose solutions.

The author and SAGE would like to thank the following reviewers for their comments during the course of the development of this book:

Biko Agozino, Virginia Tech University

Sarah Becker, Louisiana State University

Kate M. Centellas, University of Mississippi

Samuel Gerald Collins, Towson University

Erin E. Gilles, University of Southern Indiana

Dari Green, Louisiana State University

Landon Hancock, Kent State University

Julie Howenstine, University of Saint Francis

Cristina Karmas, Graceland University

David A. Kinney, Central Michigan University

David Kozak, Fort Lewis College

Anthony Kwame Harrison, Virginia Tech

Leah E. LeFebvre, University of Alabama

Tracy Walker, Virginia State University

Daniel M. Welliver, Juniata College

CHAPTER 1

ORIENTATION TO ETHNOGRAPHY AND COGNITIVE ETHNOGRAPHY

ETHNOGRAPHY

Ethnography can be defined as a social science (Aberle, 1987) research strategy that combines systematic interview and observation to characterize the way of life of a people or group. Knowledge of this way of life is known as a culture, and every human group has a culture. Defining cognitive ethnography requires adding that the whole enterprise places special emphasis on *understanding and including the language of a people with whom the work is conducted.* In earlier anthropology, this approach was also referred to as "ethnoscience." We identify with this term and refrain from using it only because it has experienced other semantic variation. This brief definition of ethnography carries with it important attributes that show how cognitive ethnography differs from other kinds of ethnography. For any ethnography, the first attribute is that it is *written.* There are indeed other media for communication of human knowledge. Examples such as motion pictures and videos come to mind. However, standing behind all these media is a written script of some sort. For most ethnography, this script is in a monograph, article, or book.

Scripts thus become the written rules, procedures, and other instructions for how individuals within a cultural group behave with and perceive one another. Ethnographers write down their own observations, their recollections, and what their consultants tell them. An ethnographer's perceptions must, whatever the media in which they are recorded, be kept separate from what the consultant communicates. Moreover, *these records must be kept separate from the very beginning of the ethnography.* Only in this way can the consultant's knowledge system be given the same opportunity for informing scientific or scholarly discourse as any other system of knowledge.

The second attribute of cognitive ethnography is that researchers rely on interview and observation but *primarily* on interview. This feature may appear counterintuitive. When a newly arrived researcher comes to a research site, the first activity he or she will undertake is observation. However, to understand the cultural knowledge of another people, both the researcher and the consultant need to develop a common communication base from which to proceed. This book favors interview over observation, particularly for beginning ethnographic research. The practical reasons are very simple. Observations, particularly of behavior in a strange place, are subject to misinterpretations over which the researchers have little or no control. Outside researchers have no control over them because they are interpreted based on the knowledge gained from their own experience. The experience often counts for very little when in a strange setting.

There are two theoretical reasons for using interviewing and language. The first reason is based on the work of the linguist Noam Chomsky (1968). He showed that all human languages share a grammatical deep structure, even though their surface grammars may differ. Based on a common deep structure, language grammars and learning follow universal patterns. Thus, all languages are, to a significant degree, intertranslatable.

The second reason revolves around the work of anthropologists Joseph Casagrande and Kenneth Hale (1967). They found that different human languages share certain semantic relationships. Through their study of the Tohono O'Odham folk definitions, they identified 13 different semantic relationships that appear to be shared among all languages. These fundamental relationships are the building blocks of cognitive anthropology's theory: *modification, taxonomy, and queuing.* Modification, or attribution, gives the listener discrete information about a term and its meaning. Taxonomy shows whether one term describes something that is a kind of something else; that is, "X is a kind of Y" or "X is a Y." Queuing, or sequence, states "X and then Y" or "X happens (or exists) and then Y." Queuing does not necessarily mean that X is a precondition of Y. A precondition denotes a more complex logical and semantic relationship, which will be discussed in Chapter 7. Taxonomy, attribution, and queuing can tie together many other, more complex semantic relationships. Together, these three relationships will be referred to in this book as MTQ schema.

Through the application of these semantic relationships in interview and analysis, ethnographers can structure written texts and discourse around the knowledge of a speaker. The result is a much deeper and richer picture of what the speaker knows. This theory can free both the ethnographer and the native consultant from certain hidden biases that reside in observation.

How Observation Is Integrated With Interview

A cautionary note is necessary. While consultants can describe much of what they do, *it is not a substitute for observation.* Reconciling what people tell a researcher versus what a researcher may observe them do requires acknowledging that *both speech and observed behavior are kinds of knowledge.* The polymath Michael Polanyi (1966) describes what people can talk about as the *explicit dimension* of knowledge. He describes the second kind of knowledge as the *tacit dimension* of knowledge—that is, the knowledge of what people do but cannot entirely explain. Both of these kinds of knowledge interact with each other: We do things; we think through how we do things; we may change how we do things. Polanyi maintained that one dimension "destroys" the other. He uses the analogy of a person typing (nowadays using a keyboard), who then thinks consciously about keying. When that happens, the performance usually ceases to function. Another example is kinesics, better known as "body language." In those cases, if people literally think about these things while they are doing them, their thinking will interfere with what they are doing. Thus, while there are certain aspects of knowledge that can be transmitted primarily through speech, demonstration, or practice, most knowledge is transmitted through a *combination* of these three. Roles such as apprenticeship exist in all societies and incorporate all these forms of instruction.

Polanyi (1966) thus famously observed that "we know more than we can tell" (p. 4). While he was focusing on knowledge transfer and apprenticeship of scientists in universities, the same generality can be expanded to social interaction in the wider human society.

How Schoepfle Became a Lender and a Borrower in Navajo Society

I was newly arrived at the Navajo reservation and was asked by a tribal employee—herself a Navajo—if she could borrow some money. I loaned her the money. In a few weeks, I asked her if she would repay the loan, because *I* needed the money. While she readily produced the money, I was surprised by the apparent look of disgust she gave me. As I worked more in the tribal office, I noticed that Navajos would often borrow money and then not repay it. Yet the lender would not refuse the request. I then changed my approach. I would never refuse a request to loan money. Whenever I needed it back, I would simply ask to borrow it. The result was more congenial. From this and similar incidents, I reasoned that borrowing or asking for a ride were expressions of support and generosity between people that was a fundamental of Navajo society and social organization. I had read about this value in books but had not experienced it. When I did not want to give somebody a ride (because I did not have the time or the gas), I would apologetically cite "car trouble." I never said "no." Non-Navajo employees, on the other hand, often made a point of collecting "debts" and felt disrespectful of Navajo borrowing practices.

Every human being is born into a group: the family of orientation. Whenever a new human group forms, members bring their past cultural knowledge with them. The family is the first of many groups that individuals join, in this case through birth, and leave behind during the course of their lives. New group members adapt to one another, define ways of life for the group, and begin to pursue goals. The new group develops knowledge that is specific to itself. This knowledge represents the beginning of a new group culture. Similar to Polanyi's (1966) formulation, it contains (1) knowledge about how things are (*knowing that*, Ryle, 1946), (2) knowledge about how to get things done (*knowing how*, Ryle, 1946), and (3) the affect, lines of friendship, or our knowledge of likes and dislikes.

Participant Observation

Learning cultural knowledge, then, involves a membership in networks or social groupings. Within this group or network, cultural knowledge is as much a process of becoming as it is a finished product. As long as a group exists, it will elaborate its own cultural knowledge. Any ethnography is thus a snapshot. A dynamic process such as the knowledge of becoming is difficult to capture. The best ethnographers can usually hope for is to describe the cultural knowledge of a group at one moment in time, what is called the "ethnographic present." Ethnographers can collect life histories or careers, and compose ethnographies through time. However, a life history is not a perfect record of the past. It *reflects how people see the past today, within the limits of their current cultural knowledge.* Thus, this book stresses the "ethnographic present" (see Sanjek, 1991).

Following Polanyi's (1966) scheme of tacit and explicit knowledge, the *formal education* of the classroom verbalizes explicit knowledge. At the other extreme is *apprenticeship*, where observed demonstration and tacit knowledge dominate. However, even in an apprenticeship, language is crucial. People ask questions; then they practice. The same is true for ethnographers, and this alternation between asking questions and observing/practicing something becomes the basis of what has been called *participant observation* in ethnography. In cognitive ethnography, participant observation becomes a form of homing process. Through this process, an individual tries to master as much of a system of knowledge as possible through alternation between observation and interview (Schoepfle, Topper, & Fisher, 1974). Then they test what they have heard and seen from their own practices as well as those of others (see Figure 1.1).

Cognitive ethnographic theory is also preferable because the fact remains that one cannot learn a culture by observing alone, any more than one can learn how to play baseball by simply watching. The experience of Oswald Werner's (1993, p. 16) first baseball game is particularly pertinent here:

> I was invited to my first baseball game and watched with interest the strangely dull game. There was a man with the

Figure 1.1 Diagram of the Participant Observation Homing Process

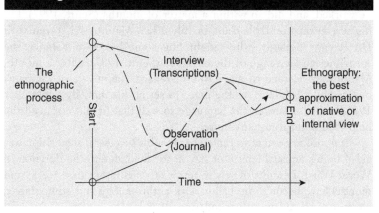

Source: Werner and Schoepfle, 1987, vol 1.

stick who tried to hit a ball that another guy threw at him. He was not very good at hitting the ball, but when he did he ran from one pillow in the grass to the next and tried to get there before the other player caught him with the ball.

Then another player hit the ball and it disappeared in the bushes behind the field. Before, the guys who hit the ball ran fast, but this player was so upset about the loss of the ball that he walked dejectedly around the square formed by the four pillows. As he came around the last bend his comrades ran up to him, shook his hand and consoled him by saying something like "don't worry about the ball, we'll pitch in and buy a new one." Soon they somehow did get a new ball and the strange game continued.

Everybody must ask, listen, observe, and try out what has been seen and heard. Observation is necessary but not sufficient. Everyone must talk to people and ask questions.

In the days of Bronislaw Malinowski, at the turn of the 20th century, participant observation was a radical departure from armchair scholarship. Armchair anthropology drew conveniently from whatever missionary, military, or traveler tales supported the argument of an author. Participant observation required ethnographers to see for themselves what was going on and conduct themselves as systematically as possible. They could no longer depend on the tales of others without verifying for themselves what was going on. Malinowski's achievement was all the more dramatic because he acquired fluency in Kilivila, the language of the Trobriand Islanders, with whom he worked, and did so within a matter of months (Senft, 1997). On his arrival on the Trobriands in July 1915, Malinowski stayed with Dr. Raynor Bellamy, who taught him some basics of Kilivila, the Austronesian language of the islanders (Senft, 1987). After a month, Malinowski decided to move to Omarakana, the village of the paramount chief To'uluwa, as the place to set up his tent. By September 1915, he had mastered the language so well that he did not need the help of an interpreter any more.

It is also important to remember that his successful acquisition was aided by his unusual length of stay in the field, due to the duration of World War I. Lengths of stay in terms of years rather than weeks and months have become the hallmark of anthropology and ethnography, albeit possibly less prevalent today.

Participant Observation and Perspective

Malinowski's participant observation introduced new challenges to this novel ethnographic research. First, when ethnographers both observe and ask questions, they will become more active participants, becoming *a part of what they are studying.* They are often there, on site, day in and day out. They get involved in what is going on. Similarly, the consultants and other people in the group change, to some extent, to accommodate the ethnographer. Ethnographers, in other words, become to some extent a part of the group and part of what they are studying.

Just how far does the ethnographer become a part of the group? There are a number of both professional and popular accounts of ethnographers "going native" (O'Reilly, 2009). When ethnographers "go native," readers often assume that the ethnographers *think* or *believe* that they have become native. "Going native" does not usually mean that they actually have acquired the natives' cultural knowledge and background (Wagner, 1975). Rather, the natives accommodate the ethnographers into their interpersonal and political lives.

The native may well tell the researcher, "You really understand us." These compliments often reflect the natives' appreciation that somebody from outside their own society respects them for who they are. They appreciate that the researcher does not try to make them change their way of life according to what some outsider wants them to be. In more recent times, anthropologists and other social scientists often arrive at sites at the behest of governmental and nongovernmental agencies. They are thus often expected to be teachers, health care practitioners, as well as ethnographers. These expectations, in turn, reflect on how the ethnographer needs to accommodate to the native ways of life. It does not mean, however, that the researcher has acquired the native mind-set.

One special case of "going native" stands out: language fluency. We outlined above, with Malinowski, how anthropologists have attained native language fluency. This fact too is well respected by the natives, and by an ethnographer's colleagues. Language fluency, however, has a special meaning: Knowledge of the language's grammar, phonology, and vocabulary is *sufficient to generate and understand meaningful utterances.* Those considered fluent in a language, however, are usually sensible enough to observe that they—as well as any nonnative in any society—will function much better when working actively with a competent bilingual/native coresearcher.

MATERIAL CULTURE AND CULTURAL DURABILITY

A related question arises regarding material culture and how it relates to the definition of ethnography and culture. I address this question by asking, "How do you use the right tool for the right job?" Answering that question without asking the users can create problems particularly in archaeology, where the people who may have used the tools or implements in a site are no longer available for interviewing. Archaeologists thus have no recent knowledgeable source for conducting ethnography. They have to depend on historical reconstruction by natives, maybe comparing with other sites or inferring from elsewhere, where such information is available.

Ethnography needs to ask how durable is culture. Behavior is ephemeral. One possibility is for it simply to reside in memory, where it can later be recalled. However, this solution raises issues of the *systematic distortion hypothesis* (Shweder and D'Andrade 1980). More useful for the preservation of behavior are texts, photographs, strips of film, or various kinds of digital recordings. All of these represent products of behavior, or artifacts. A text is a record of a native utterance. Figure 1.2 helps to show the interrelationships among cultural knowledge, ephemeral behavior, and texts.

Figure 1.2 Cultural Knowledge, Ephemeral Behavior, and Texts

CULTURAL KNOWLEDGE
Memory accessible through language

Feedback Loop

EPHEMERAL BEHAVIOR

CHANCE AND/OR NOISE – THE ENVIRONMENT

Feedback Loop

RESULTS OF BEHAVIOR
artifacts, also texts

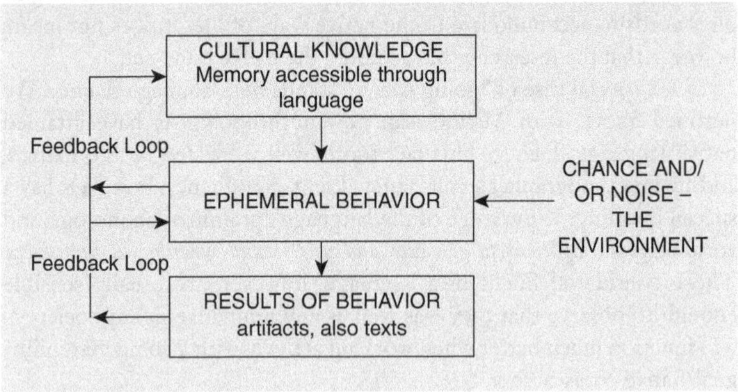

Source: Werner and Schoepfle (1987a).

The completeness of a cultural description also needs to be considered. Anthropologists such as Michael Agar have raised the question of what happens when anthropologists describe only parts of a people's way of life and culture. He termed this research "ethnographic," for describing some of the knowledge shared by a group of people. His question is important, and this book uses both "ethnographic" and "ethnography."

KINDS OF ETHNOGRAPHY

A distantly related question is "Is all culture describable?" This book has noted that culture can be seen as a group of people's knowledge of learned behavior, artifacts, social relationships, politics, religion, and the economy. Anthropologists have described culture as pertaining to all of humanity, to groups, and to parts of an individual's psychological makeup. This issue was summarized by the oft-quoted phrase attributed to anthropologist Clyde Kluckhohn and psychologist Henry Murray (1953): "Every man is in certain respects like all other men, like some other men, like no other man." The inverted pyramid in Figure 1.3 illustrates the variability of groups and how they can be studied.

Figure 1.3 Range of Cultures and Methods of Describing Them

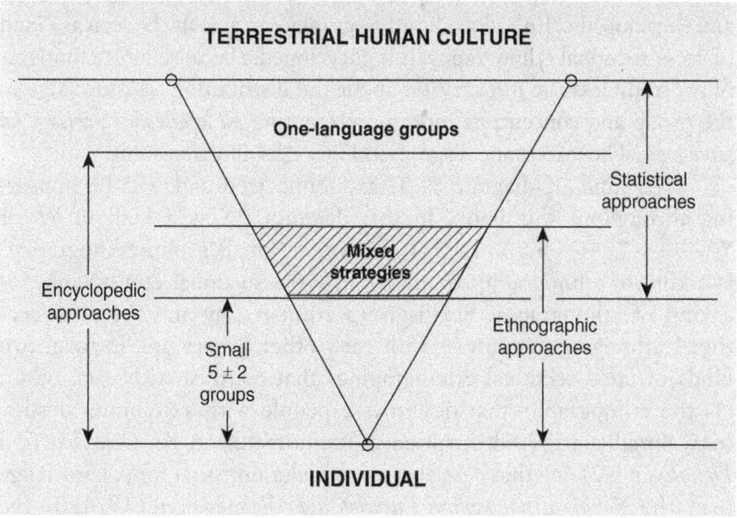

Source: Werner and Schoepfle (1987a).

Starting at the bottom, the first kind of ethnography describes small groups with memberships ranging from three to seven people. These groups are the subject of ethnography *par excellence*. The second kind of ethnography is *cross-sectional ethnography*, of which there are two types. One describes a cross-section of *people*, the other a cross section of *knowledge*. In describing a cross section of people, ethnographers look at human beings who share a common history or destiny. James Spradley wrote *You Owe Yourself a Drunk* (1970), which describes the lifeways of the Skid Row homeless in Seattle, Washington. However, Spradley did not study them as an interacting human group or groups but rather as a cross section of homeless people. Assumed here is that all these people face similar problems and could be seen as having a common destiny. See Agar's book *Ripping and Running* (1974) for a similar description of drug addic ts.

The third kind of cross-sectional ethnography is the encyclopedic. It is intended to study and describe as completely as possible the cultural knowledge base of a domain such as agriculture, child rearing, or warfare. Examples include the encyclopedias of Western civilization, the *Encyclopedia Bororo* (Albisetti & Venturelli, 1962), and the Navajo ethnologic dictionary (Franciscan Fathers, 2015). Others concentrate on selected domains, such as the Navajo knowledge of health and medicine in the *Navajo Ethnomedical Encyclopedia* (Werner et al., 1976) and Harold Conklin's (1983) *Ethnographic Atlas of Ifugao*.

Most ethnographies are mixtures of all three—group, cross-sectional, and encyclopedic. Encyclopedic ethnography can actually be seen as a kind of cross-sectional ethnography. It is encyclopedic because most ethnographers study less the information about the distribution of knowledge in the group and concentrate more on presenting *all available knowledge on some topic*. The taxonomic diagram in Figure 1.4 illustrates this.

This kind of diagram is a taxonomic tree and will be appearing throughout this book. In this diagram, "X is a kind of Y," or **Y** o——— T ———▸o **X**. In this diagram, a "small-group ethnography" is a kind of ethnography. Similarly, a "cross-sectional ethnography" is a kind of ethnography. Small-group ethnography and the cross-sectional ethnography contrast with each other. There are, in turn, two kinds of cross-sectional ethnographies that contrast with each other: (1) the ethnography that describes a people with a common destiny (e.g., Spradley's 1970 description of the homeless in *You Owe Yourself a Drunk*) and (2) one that describes a particular domain of folk knowledge (e.g., the *Navajo Ethnomedical Encyclopedia*, Werner et al., 1976). In the basic description of ethnography discussed so far, this book does not

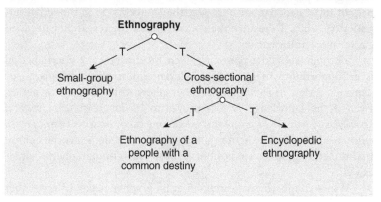

Figure 1.4   Kinds of Ethnography

Ethnography

Small-group ethnography

Cross-sectional ethnography

Ethnography of a people with a common destiny

Encyclopedic ethnography

Source: Werner and Schoepfle (1987a).

specify the size or the complexity of the group. Instead, it selects the term "group" rather than relying on terms such as "tribe," "band," or "ethnic group" because ethnography does not limit itself by how large or small the so-called group should be.

ABDUCTIVE REASONING IN COGNITIVE ETHNOGRAPHY

Cognitive ethnography is indeed a social science research strategy, but a special one. It is not *deductive*: Researchers in ethnography do not formulate broad theory about the human condition and test specific hypotheses through experimentation. It is also not *inductive*: Ethnographers do not derive broad generalizations about observed patterns from a limited number of observations and test them on a broader sample. Instead, it is what Agar (2006, 2010) called *abductive*. That is, ethnography encounters contradictions in incomplete data and generates explanations to resolve them. Agar refers to these contradictions as "breakdowns." These breakdowns are a form of "epistemological window" (Werner & Schoepfle, 1987b). They are opportunities to learn something new and unexpected. For example, it is very healthy for ethnographers to ask themselves, "Why do two consultants contradict each other?" In crediting the 19th-century philosopher of science Charles Sanders Peirce, Michael Agar (2010) summarized that this abductive reasoning "calls for taking surprises seriously and creating new concepts to account for them. No more tossing the problem into error variance. No more testing the goodness of fit of new data against available concepts, as in inductive statistics" (p. 289). To resolve the contradiction, the researcher needs to gather more information.

Through abductive reasoning, then, inconsistency or contradiction is an opportunity to gain more relevant information. Inconsistency demands a view of something ethnographers would not see or notice. Even if the knowledge system proves to be inconsistent, *a cultural knowledge system can be assumed valid and internally consistent until proven otherwise.* Failure to promote this stance not only demeans the culture that the ethnographer studies but demeans the ethnographer's culture as well.

When conducting research, an ethnographer needs to remember that it is a *social enterprise* that cannot be conducted by one person. At the least, the social cooperation includes the researcher and the people with whom the research is conducted. Those with whom the research is conducted are not "subjects." The term "research subjects" pertains to isolated individuals who are supposed to be affected by the researcher only as part of an experiment (Sieber & Tolich, 2013). Ethnographic description is coproduced by the ethnographers and the people with whom they work. As a group, they are called "natives"; as individuals, we refer to them as "consultants." Native people are the experts in their cultural lives. As experts, they can be considered as consultants. This term thus replaces terms such as "informant" that were used by earlier anthropologists.

Ethnography is thus an *alliance* between the ethnographers and the natives (Bohannan et al., 1974). As an alliance, ethnographers *must*

1. share their own backgrounds with their native hosts as much as they might expect to obtain information about them;

2. be honest with those with whom a researcher must work;

3. negotiate carefully, and honestly, the roles of researcher and participant through time;

4. maximize interview privacy, comfort, and safety for both the native and the interviewer and balance them with the opportunity to interview and observe; and

5. consider the natives with whom they work as consultants who are expert in their cultural knowledge.

HOW ETHNOGRAPHY DIFFERS
FROM JOURNALISM

It is easy to confuse journalism and ethnography. Both may involve fieldwork and interviewing, and thus overlap in the way fieldwork is conducted. When not acting as a propaganda instrument or extreme advocacy organization, both adhere to high ethical standards of accuracy and treatment of those with whom journalists or ethnographers work. There are three important differences, however, that must be acknowledged. First, journalism tends to concentrate on the newsworthy and the special, what is often referred to as the unusual, or "man bites dog," stories. Ethnography describes in detail the everyday, or "dog bites man," stories. Stated yet another way, ethnography concentrates on what Malinowski (1922) referred to as "the *imponderabilia* of everyday life."

Second, journalism tends to highlight the activities and achievements of individuals and the changes they bring to life around them. Those interviewed by a journalist are often aware of this fact. While ethnographers may carefully note these events and the individuals involved in them, the differences in emphasis are important.

Third, journalists tend to depend far more than ethnographers on observation (see Lubet, 2018). In journalism, such a stance may be reasonable because, first, there is often very little time to prepare a feature article or report. For journalism, lengthy interviewing and analysis might therefore be considered overly time-consuming, in light of the information they feel they are receiving and must transmit to the public. The result may be the inadvertent blending of dramatic fiction for information (see Cooke, 1980; Lubet, 2018) critique.

More important is that journalists are going to depend more on observation because they often share more of the culture of the people with whom they are researching. Ethnographers, however, acknowledge that doing research with groups with a similar culture and language to theirs can actually be more treacherous. This is because they may not notice where they have misjudged a situation. Ironically, some of the best examples of thoroughness in such investigations come from journalists. For good examples of care and precision in reporting, see Jon Krakauer's coverage of Christopher McCandless's fatal travails in *Into the Wild* (1996), his portrayal of the experiences of Mount Everest climbers in *Into Thin Air* (1999), and his description of the Church of Jesus Christ of Latter-Day Saints in his book *Under the Banner of Heaven* (2003). All involved considerable written response to peer review and debate with the families and official organizations involved.

EVERYONE IS BIASED AND MUST COPE WITH THE FACT

Ethnographers in the past have used a number of devices for controlling their biases. The late Robert Redfield (1930) recommended that all ethnographers should come clean and talk about their biases. He noted, for example, that he maintained a strong bias favoring the underdog. This is a common bias among ethnographers and perhaps one reason why they tend to study "down" rather than "up" (Nader, 1969).

Relatively few anthropologists have worked with people whose status, income, or prestige is higher than their own. Until recently, the most common status for anthropologists or ethnographers has been that of the university professor. It is safe to assume that most American ethnographers are either in, or aspire to become part of, the upper-middle-class "intelligentsia." Laura Nader (1969) wrote an article that has become almost a manifesto, calling for more ethnographic work on the upper classes, top executives, politicians, and other people who are "above" the ethnographers in U.S. society.

Recent fieldwork has responded, with studies such as those by Karen Ho (2009), who conducted an ethnographic study of Wall Street investment bankers' institutional culture from February 1998 through June 1999. Her primary source for participant observation was on-the-job.

In any event, it is difficult for an ethnographer to be aware of these biases, and the difficulty becomes greater the more similar the culture of the native consultant is to that of the ethnographer. Ethnography has three principal defenses that reduce or mitigate bias. The first is through the systematic application of methodologies for interviews, observation, and documentary analysis. This book will show that interviews are structured around the knowledge of the consultant, not dependent on a preconceived set of questions. This form of interview structure will help the ethnographer to understand the knowledge of another culture in as nonjudgmental and unbiased a way as possible.

Subsequent chapters will explain in greater detail how a cognitive ethnography begins with an open-ended or "grand tour" question. The ethnographer has to negotiate this question carefully with the consultant, to make sure that both are addressing the same subject domain. The interview records the terms and phrases given by the consultant, and the ethnographer develops follow-up questions from them. These follow-up questions are based on the three theoretically universal semantic relationships mentioned earlier: modification, taxonomy, and queuing. The process is thus highly structured. Answers to the interview questions can be generated and combined to denote elaborate relationships of causality or precondition. While the answers can be complex, both the interviewer and the consultant can better track what each other is thinking or wants to find out.

A second defense relies on multiple sources. That is, ethnographers try to work with more than one consultant from different backgrounds. They also compare what these different consultants tell them with what they observe and with the documentary sources they find. By using all these sources, ethnographers attempt to pull together a structured, consistent description of the culture.

A third defense is to plan and report thoroughly on one's research. As in other social sciences, cognitive ethnographers prepare for their research as thoroughly as possible before conducting interviews and observation. When they write a final report or description, they carefully note and outline the limitations of their studies by describing who they interviewed, where and what settings they observed, and the kinds of documentation they examined. In this fashion, future ethnographers can hopefully discover limitations and compensate for them.

Avoiding Bias Is a Methodological, Not a Moral or Ethical, Stance

Everyone has biases, and they must be dealt with. Refusal to deal with them renders one *ethnocentric*. This refusal can emerge through sloth or through ideological blinders. Either source is pernicious because it leads to an ill-informed judgment of a group's way of life. Ethnographers arrive at judgments only after they have exhausted all available means of further description. Avoiding bias is thus an *operational* or *methodological* stance (Bidney, 1967), not a moral or ethical one.

Cultural relativism's original intent was to establish that one should not judge any culture, or cultural knowledge system, as better than as or worse than any other (Benedict, 1959). This stance also does not mean that "anything goes" (c.f. Bruner, 1990). It is a methodological and epistemological stance, not a moral or ethical one. This stance, in turn, indicates how the ethnographic record should be kept. A researcher must ask how a cultural practice or belief works, rather than prejudging it. It also requires the researcher to maintain an egalitarian relationship with the consultants with whom they conduct research. They must treat all these people as having rights to the same quality, rigor, and intellectual honesty that ethnographers would pursue for social inquiry in their own society.

Ethnographers also need to describe the power relationships in a given society, as well as associated histories of colonialism, slavery, or warfare. Writings of this kind of knowledge may result in contested histories and may require acknowledgment that sometimes one has been telling the story from only one viewpoint. These power relationships must be dealt with descriptively and without taking sides, particularly during the conduct of the research.

Finally, the ethnographer accomplishes little by denigrating his or her culture. Such denigration is as pernicious as ethnocentrism. Western civilization and the United States, for example, have both served as exemplars of greed, duplicity, and brutality, to name a few well-deserved labels. It is possible also that these faults have bled over into the social theory of social scientists, philosophers, or historians. Overrepresenting these faults and doubts through overreliance on self-criticism succeeds in paralyzing fieldwork and research.

PREPARATION FOR AN ETHNOGRAPHER'S CAREER: ETHNOGRAPHER AS EXPERT WITNESS

No matter the social science discipline, the ethnographer may have to report findings to governmental agencies or testify before the courts. That is, they may be asked to be *expert witnesses* (Rosen, 1977). Until 1993, the Frye General Acceptance standard prevailed (*Frye v. United States*, 1923). That is, an individual's admissibility of their expert witness testimony depended on its being "*sufficiently established to have gained general acceptance in the particular field in which it belongs*" (italics added). With *Daubert v. Merrell Dow Pharmaceuticals, Inc.* (1993), the U.S. Supreme Court superseded the Frye General Acceptance standard with the *Federal Rules of Evidence* (Pub. L. No. 93-595; National Court Rules Committee, 2021), which Congress subsequently passed as legislation on January 2, 1975. The *Federal Rules of Evidence* govern the introduction of evidence at civil and criminal trials in the U.S. federal trial courts. They are amended annually by the Supreme Court.

The *Federal Rules of Evidence* are recognized by the Supreme Court as the law. The changes to jurisprudence were substantial. First, the judges in a federal court now were "to *assume the obligation* as well as *exercise the discretion* to evaluate admission of expert witnesses." They were also to do so at the outset of the trial. The court thus becomes the gatekeeper of the evidence. With *Daubert* (1993), the emphasis shifted *from* deciding how well received the theory or the individual testifying is *to* assessing the validity of the evidence in support of the testimony. Section 702 of the *Federal Rules of Evidence* is the part most often cited. This rule states,

> A witness who is qualified as an expert by knowledge, skill, experience, training, or education may testify in the form of an opinion or otherwise if:
>
> (a)　the expert's scientific, technical or other specialized knowledge will help the trier of fact to understand the evidence or to determine a fact in issue;
>
> (b)　the testimony is based on sufficient facts or data;
>
> (c)　the testimony is the product of reliable principles and methods; and
>
> (d)　the expert has reliably applied the principles and methods to the facts of the case (National Court Rules Committee, 2021)

These four criteria also form the basis of a so-called Daubert motion, a motion that is raised before or during a trial to exclude the presentation of unqualified evidence to the jury. The argument can exclude the testimony of an expert witness if the witness's testimony is found to be insufficient or the methods used to obtain data are questionable.

Section 705 of the *Federal Rules of Evidence* becomes important regarding dissemination of data:

> Unless the court orders otherwise, an expert may state an opinion—and give the reasons for it—without first testifying to the underlying facts or data. *But the expert may be required to disclose these facts or data on cross-examination.* (National Court Rules Committee, 2021; italics added)

In other words, ethnographers may not have to produce all of their data at trial but may have to produce them when demanded on Discovery ("pretrial procedures providing for the exchange of information between the parties involved in the proceedings," Brittanica.com, n.d.) by the opposing side. Any aspiring ethnographer is urged to read Sections 703 (Bases of an Expert's Opinion Testimony), 704 (Opinion on an Ultimate Issue), 705 (Disclosing the Facts or Data Underlying an Expert's Opinion), and 706 (Court-Appointed Expert Witnesses).

Ethnographers are also urged to sort out what they are being told by other sources about events. Achieving a full understanding of a consultant's knowledge does not always mean complete acceptance. To record accurate information, an ethnographer needs to take into consideration questions of who, what, where, when, antecedents, and consequents. In other words, they must answer these questions:

1. What exactly happened?

2. Who exactly was involved in this event?

3. Where did this event happen?

4. When did this event happen?

5. What were the antecedents and consequents of this event?

In addition to better data being included in their research, ethnographers will have either the opportunity or the obligation to serve as expert witnesses (Campbell et al., 2017). Because of *Daubert* (1993), an expert witness may need to have done research directly relevant to the trial. Leila Rodriguez (2014) recounted the methodological and ethical issues she faced when she did fieldwork and analysis for a defendant's defense team. She ultimately avoided a "battle of experts" because the defendant accepted a plea deal that amended his charges to a less serious offense. Nevertheless, the stakes were high considering that the individual charged would face possible prison time.

Finally, ethnographers must be prepared to understand what is expected of them for protecting the privacy of the consultants and fellow researchers. Considerable debate has gone on throughout the American Anthropological Association (AAA) on how to protect both privacy and anonymity. A definitive discussion on the subject is beyond the scope of this book. It is one of the reasons, however, why this book stresses the need to understand the laws of privacy and confidentiality applicable directly to the nations, communities, and people with whom we are to conduct the research. Laws obviously differ from place to place, and a good background acquired in one place may or may not transfer to another. It may, however, serve as a good basis for comparison. See Chapter 2 for more details.

PLANNING AND PROPOSING A RESEARCH PROJECT

E thnographers must have a plan formulated before entering the field. They will need it not only for a reminder but also to consult in the event of having to make changes in plans during the research. Flexibility is thus paramount, but it is not equivalent to "free-wheeling." There is a need, in turn, for transparency in all forms of the research operation toward the project sponsor, the people with whom the ethnographer works in the field, and other agencies who claim a stakeholder interest. In short, all efforts need to be made to turn the unexpected into either a research opportunity or at least a containable emergency.

Planning for research is best illustrated by the seemingly contradictory statement attributed to Dwight D. Eisenhower that "plans are worthless; planning is everything." Ethnographers will conclude that the best research plan will survive up to the beginning of the fieldwork. They will at the same time need to recognize that they are lost if they do not have a plan to start with.

The basics of research plans answer the questions of *what* subject is to be studied, *where* the study takes place, with *whom* the study is conducted, and *when* the study is best conducted. Answers to these questions become the plans that will be the basis of the proposal. Proposals need to link theory, the researcher's specific questions, and the data collection that will best address the questions.

THE PROPOSAL

A proposal is a document that prospective ethnographers write before they get into the field. During the ethnographic process, it should be consulted often. A good proposal combines the best features of a map and a compass. It tells ethnographers where they are, in addition to where they want to be, and highlights likely paths that show how to get there. Once in the field, ethnographers are surrounded by the riches of human culture, and therefore of ethnographic data. Virtually all new ethnographers have discovered that it is easy to lose one's way and chase after exotic but irrelevant detail. The following discusses the minimum attributes that a research proposal might take, in light of the practical research issues confronting all ethnographers.

What the Ethnographer Will Study

This section of the proposal contains the research problem statement and a review of previous work in the subject area. It includes the literature review, which in turn includes a review of theories. Such theories are a form of conceptual guidance that has been applied to similar problems in the past. In the best of all possible worlds, it should include a new theoretical synthesis—a better way of looking at the problem. A word of caution is necessary, however: a literature review can become lengthy. Often the bulk of it can be put in an appendix. The proposal proper should include only some form of summary—at most about 10 pages—of a lengthy literature review.

Sometimes ethnographers may want simply to describe as much of the culture as possible. This sentiment applies particularly at the beginning of the research. Later on, the researcher may find that other theoretical issues emerge that affect the research. Much theory can be derived from disciplines such as psychology, economics, political science, and sociology. To various degrees, ethnographic research can inform the explanatory power of these theories in turn.

When and for How Long the Research Is Conducted

Every ethnography is a compromise between stated goals and the time available in which to meet them. One of the most common mistakes that ethnographers make is underestimating the time required for the work to be done. The question of *when* depends on factors peculiar to the situation the researcher will be studying. Some circumstances are frequent, while some circumstances are infrequent and may happen rarely. A researcher may wish to avoid major events such as natural disasters, revolutions, national elections, or wars. Although they are doubtless interesting sources of information, ethnography concentrates more on the everyday, unlike the reporting tendencies within journalism (see Chapter 1).

Before setting up a schedule, the proposal must discuss the length of stay in the field, which forces questions such as how researchers expect their project to progress through the weeks or months of research. The proposal also addresses the time to be taken for preparation, establishing contact, transporting/commuting, interviewing, observation, transcription of interviews, managing the database, analysis in the field, and perhaps even some report writing in the field.

Where the Ethnographer Is Personally Located

Two questions of "where" involve both questions of where the research will be conducted and where the researcher will be living. Answers to both of these questions involve extensive background research in geography, climate, politics, foreign affairs, and anything else that would be relevant to the research conditions. Regarding the location of the research, there are four different kinds of interview locations: the white room, the grass hut, the muddy field, and the commute. The term "white room" means that the interview is sequestered in a room far away from the usual field of activities. The setting may distort the kinds of information an interviewer may receive, and close the researchers off from observing what is going on around them. On the other hand, there are advantages. One advantage was illustrated in interviews conducted in some New Mexico villages. The interviews included finding out why local people would travel to a clinic located farther away from the ones in their own village. It soon became clear that people from the local village were predictably reluctant even to visit clinics, much less to talk about socially transmitted diseases, because they were afraid that their neighbors or relatives would conclude the worst about them. Instead, they would drive to a clinic 40 or 50 miles away, where they were less known. Under these circumstances, the white room interview elicited better results.

In the 1920s, Leslie White conducted several ethnographies of the Rio Grande Pueblo Indian villages by interviewing individuals off-site. The Indians were very secretive. Most of us today would consider such sequestering ethically dubious. However, in the 1920s, few people had such qualms and admired White for having "beat the system" of Pueblo secrecy, especially since it was "in the name of science." Future generations of Pueblo Indians will continue to judge if the deception was worthwhile.

A second kind of interview setting is the grass hut. Here, the interviewer moves closer to where the social interaction is actually taking place, but it is not necessarily the site of that interaction. When the

Nuer in Nigeria allowed Edward Evans-Pritchard to pitch his tent in the middle of their village, that arrangement was grass hut living. Interviewing under a tree outside the native village is an almost prototypical case in anthropology. The obvious advantage of the grass hut interview is that a consultant can point to, demonstrate, and enlist other people to help illustrate something.

A third kind of interview setting is what Werner called the "muddy field." Werner used this label when describing the work of Christina Gladwin and her decision-making studies of African, Mexican, and Guatemalan farmers (see Gladwin, 1989). She would watch them while they were planting, cultivating, irrigating, or fertilizing their corn. She would then ask them about what they were doing at the same time they were conducting these activities. In these cases, some of these activities appeared so automatic that it was otherwise difficult to discuss them away from the immediate context in which they were observed. A large number of the decision-making studies seem to fall in this category. Thus, the muddy field was exceedingly valuable in collecting detailed decision-making information.

A fourth, more recent interview setting is the commuter or part-time interview. For example, in the Navajo reservation school ethnographies (Werner et al., 1976), the ethnographers would reside somewhere in a nearby administrative center or town, commute to the school daily while it was in session, and return to their accommodations at night. This approach has been especially useful in rapid-assessment research. Here, the interview is only a part of the overall enterprise, and often little time is available to conduct it (Beebe, 2001).

The commuter setting also becomes important for longer-term research in areas considered too dangerous to implement the other approaches. Throughout the world, recent times have seen an increase in violence due to warfare (Kilcullen, 2010) between nations, insurgencies and counterinsurgencies within natioins (Kilcullen, 2010), ongoing battles between states and crime syndicates (Kilcullen, 2013), or a high crime rate. Anthropologists have been discouraged from conducting research in some areas, and they themselves have often decided to avoid staying in them (Wladyka & Yaworsky, 2017). The commuter setting has become a resort in circumstances where ethnographers need to stay out of the way of danger.

Considerations of *where* also involve questions such as whether the site is situated in a rural area, a small urban area, or a large metropolitan port. Crosscutting these questions are those pertaining to climate. For example, is the research to be conducted in a humid, humid subtropical, temperate, high desert, hot desert, arctic, subarctic, or boreal forest environment? In all these circumstances, ethnographers need to know about the availability of water, electricity, transportation, and housing. Safety again emerges as an issue. As a general rule, ethnographers first make contact and then bring all their gear after someone has offered them safe housing. It is rare that ethnographers are parachuted into the hosts' territory and then face for the first time a bunch of curious strangers. The author knows only of Jean Briggs, who arrived at an Eskimo village by seaplane, apparently without prior contact. The plane took off, and she sat there on the shore of a lake with her bags until a kind native took her in. This tactic of field entry is very surprising and very dangerous, particularly where survival without a supportive family and safe shelter is impossible (J. Briggs, 1970; J. L. Briggs, 1970).

Finally, there is no guarantee that all hosts would be as generous as that Eskimo family—who concluded that someone had to take her in or she would perish. However, for "studying up" with the politically powerful or high-status groups, there may be an intake system already established through which the ethnographer must proceed (Ho, 2009). Ho (2009) found this intake system necessary to negotiate before studying stockbrokers.

The Dominant Language Researchers Will Be Speaking

As discussed in Chapter 1, command of the native language is exceedingly important. However, there are two problems with achieving this standard. First, it is not always easy to determine fluency in a second language before entering the field. As discussed in Chapter 1, any language or culture will be filtered through the system within which the researcher grew up. All ethnographers have not only a linguistic accent but also a cultural accent. Moreover, even if ethnographers are fluent in the second language, it is often convenient for them to speak to a consultant through an interpreter. Even if researchers are confident in their fluency in the native language, having an interpreter can buy time by allowing the ethnographer to pause in answering a consultant's question. The cost of hiring interpreters, in addition to the native core-searchers, needs to be factored into the proposal.

Although some researchers are not confident in their native language fluency, they can maintain control over the reliability of the transcriptions and the overall validity of the analysis. This control can be achieved through ethnographic analysis, which will be the subject of Chapters 4 to 7. The native research partners are very important.

They need to be trained, if necessary, in the transcription of their native language. Only then can outside researchers and native coresearchers work together to translate and analyze these transcriptions in a way that guarantees that all are "on the same page." Translation training has to be factored into the training of native researchers.

One principal rule or outlook is to learn as much of the native language as possible. Having stated this, the requirements of learning a language are quite daunting. They are not impossible to meet, however, and ethnographers should get as far along the path to fluency as they can. Indeed, ethnography is possible without fluency *if* the data management proceeds with care. Ethnographers have at their disposal useful resources. Some of the native consultants with whom the ethnographer works may have knowledge of English, or whatever the ethnographer's dominant language is, and may even be literate in that language. It may thus be possible for the ethnographer to teach them literacy in their own language if they do not have that skill already. Once they are biliterate, they can provide translated texts for the ethnographer to monitor and to begin schematic analysis. A feedback process is the result. The ethnographer's initial analyses of the translated texts become the beginning of a research partnership or collaboration. This practical learning process provides the partners an opportunity to become more active in the analytical process too. Thus, while such early quality control must be conducted painstakingly and slowly, both the ethnographer and the native coresearchers can learn each other's language to a level that is sufficient to proceed with the analysis. However, this system takes time and funding, and progress must be factored in as the research proceeds.

It may be tempting to ask why ethnographers need to waste time and research money in developing any foreign language competency at all, particularly if time is short and the only payoff appears to be making ethnographers vulnerable to ridicule. Here are some of the reasons. First, natives often do appreciate the effort to learn their language and are surprisingly forgiving of imperfections. It is possible that some natives express impatience at language-learning attempts because the outsiders are seen as not making a sincere effort. Natives are often generally experienced enough to tell the difference between a systematic and sincere effort and one that is not. Second, ethnographers should not confuse mistakes they find embarrassing (which are often hilarious to the natives) as native rejection. Ethnographers should thus not be discouraged when the learning attempt appears boring to both themselves and the native. Important ethnographic information is always to be found in determining how to avoid mistakes, minimize the risk of embarrassment, and make bearable the boring repetition often involved in instruction. Mistakes, in other words, can be yet another window of opportunity. Even if ethnographers cannot master the target language, they can at least get further along than they might have anticipated. When in doubt, the benefits likely exceed the costs of slow progress. Besides, "down time" or idle moments are best put to use.

Equipment for Data Gathering, Management, and Storage

Before even beginning this discussion, the paramount principle of data gathering, storage, and management must be made explicit: the *separate storage* of (a) the text data gathered directly from the consultants through interviews and (b) the observations and impressions of the ethnographer. The research budget will have to allow for the necessary equipment. In some situations, ethnographers may already own some of this equipment, having either bought it for themselves or received it from earlier project grants. If not, equipment cost needs to be factored into either the budget or the ethnographers' personal finances.

The first two obvious pieces of equipment are sound recorders and cameras. Inexperienced ethnographers often purchase or borrow a digital camera or recorder just immediately before they depart for the field. This last-minute preparation may be forced on them due to delayed financial support or procrastination. In any event, *equipment should be second nature to ethnographers by the time they depart for the field.* Even when there is electricity available it is advisable to bring batteries. In fact, bring lots of batteries. Many houses or buildings throughout the world do not have any electricity. Where they do, appropriate outlets may not be available or may be located in areas which are difficult to access, such as a floor during an interview. It is also important to make sure that the batteries are fresh and tested before use. Similarly, one needs to glance at the recorder during an interview to make sure that it is operating properly. A researcher's fumbling with technology distracts the consultant from thinking about what needs to be discussed in an interview. Difficulty using equipment properly may also adversely affect the consultant's respect for the researcher's preparation.

An associated issue involves cameras and video recorders. Some ethnographers in the past have been shy about taking pictures. Once they return home, they then regret that they did not take more pictures. The best approach is to ask the natives with whom the ethnographer works when and when not to take pictures. Ethnographers may find that the natives are perfectly happy to have their pictures taken—at the right time. They may indeed insist on being photographed, and nowadays they are likely to take pictures of the ethnographer with their own smartphones. Once the ethnographers know where, when, and with whom they can take pictures, it is best to take pictures of anything and everything. Modern smartphones allow easy indoor and outdoor shots, portraits and full-length photos, as well as candid and posed pictures. Care must be taken to make sure the subject is comfortable.

Increasingly popular in recent times is the use of smartphones for recording documents. Whether working at the National Archives or somewhere in the field, the researcher should be proficient at photographing documents (where and when permitted) and in other ways exploring the strengths and limitations of the devices being used. Before leaving for the field, the researcher should take pictures at high noon, at sunset, in the middle of the night, and any other time one might expect to be taking pictures. Ethnographers need to know what to do in any number of lighting conditions. In addition to using smartphones as cameras, consideration should be given to their use as video recorders. The advantages of being able to video record an interview are obvious. The researcher can gain information on nonlinguistic properties such as the speaker's body language and expressions, the surroundings, and the effects of other people being in the vicinity of the interview, all of which become easier to note during interview analysis. iPhones can now be used for both audio and video recording. The authors have found them useful, and they recommend, first, that when conducting an interview the smartphone should

1. *not* be handheld but should be placed on some kind of stand or other arrangement, comfortably at head height;

2. be placed so that the interviewer and the consultant are otherwise free to interact with each other, without having to hold the phone (or have it held) in one's face; and

3. be positioned in a way that distorts as little as possible the faces of the interviewer and the interviewee.

iPhones need to be tested before and after an interview. The interviewer needs to know how well and at what range the video and audio components pick up sight and sound. Similarly, if redundantly, the interviewer needs either to recharge batteries or to replace dead batteries. The authors are not aware of any technical solutions to the issues of battery power and life but await future developments. In short, the authors recommend getting a good video camera and relying on smartphones as backups. For those initiating small-scale projects close to home, iPhones may be sufficient.

Also needed are word-processing and data storage applications that allow the interviewer to store text files in a widely readable format, such as *.doc, *.docx, *.TXT, or other similar format. This requirement brings up the question of the kind of computer needed. Advances in portability, power, and memory make it almost mandatory to bring computers with adequate amounts of memory. This book makes no brand-specific recommendations on word processing, but the authors have successfully taken MS Word almost everywhere. Software is available that provides a platform for various fonts and characters. Some of it is in the public domain and is free, but it is best to purchase something that is reliable.

At the risk of exposing the age of the writer for all to see, I observe that most ethnographers are going to need to bring notebooks or the digital equivalent—lots of them. Notebooks, in some form, have important implications for data gathering as well as social interaction. Not only will a notebook help record information, it can actually become an integral part of the interview itself. I refer to some sort of pad that is easily portable but not too small to hold information—such as stenographer's pads. The notebook can be either electronic or paper. Once the interview begins, the interviewer may be writing furiously.

After the interviews are finished, the information obtained from them will have to be stored in a secure location. With increasing numbers of younger people no longer educated in cursive writing, new equivalents for notebooks may need to be found. I welcome any information on how to deal with this educational transformation.

Along with notebooks, there may always be times when using any kind of sound or visual recording may make people uncomfortable. However, these occasions are not as frequent as many beginning ethnographers fear. In fact, I have found myself berated by those I intended to interview when I did not bring voice recorders. The reasons given were the same, whether the speaker was a Navajo living in a hogan, a county or regional planner, a rancher, or an urban-neighborhood resident: *People being interviewed consider what they have to say to be important.* If interviewers show up to an interview without the proper equipment, it may imply to the would-be consultant that they do not really consider their knowledge to be important. Obviously there will be times when speakers may be hesitant about being recorded. At other times, the interviews are not formal but may be a part of less formal conversations. Under those circumstances, the researcher needs to ask permission and ascertain what the native concerns about recording may be.

Hardware for data storage is paramount. Most storage is for interview sound recordings, interview text data, text data for personal journals, possible personal journal sound recording, and files for pictures. Additional separate hard drives for backups are recommended for all of these. Nothing is more heart wrenching than losing data. With that kind of worry in mind, it is also wise to have two backups—one for on-site, the other sent periodically off-site. Stories of anthropologists losing data on the flight home are no longer an excuse for not having the data available.

All these media require storage as well as routine backup. At least each day, the contents of the digital recorder, camera, or iPhone need to be copied or moved to a separate computer. While the requirement is indisputable, the means to achieve it vary. For example, many might recommend use of the cloud. We find ourselves in no position to recommend computer capabilities. Once the interviews are recorded and transcribed, setting up a text data system can become rather involved. Basically, any management system needs to access hard and digital data. Many times, during an interview, both will be collected. Both must be redundant, secure, and readily accessible. "Redundant" means that there should be at least two recordings of each interview in the database. In most cases, this means simply copying memory clips or cards to the hard drive or the portable remote hard drive of a computer. In addition, it is easy to expect that photographs, paper documents, and other nondigital materials will be made available to a researcher in the field. These must be stored; they are often copied on-site and stored safely on-site. Also, arrangements need to be made to transport these data copies back to the university, the agency office, or the private home of the researcher. With the advent of the cloud, data storage can, on the one hand, be easier and more secure. On the other, care must be taken to maintain security and backups, should there be failures in Cloud management or data hacks. The authors lack sufficient information to make judgments or recommendations. They therefore raise the question.

For longer stays in the field, it may be necessary to generate hardcopy to analyze interviews. The documentation generated by such analysis also needs to be stored securely. There is nothing that will invite disaster more than the people with whom the research is being conducted witnessing or reading partial documentation or analysis. These tracts can easily lead to misunderstanding, from which the researcher may at best only partially recover. Text data management must allow indexing.

Data Management for Analysis

Every ethnographic project needs a text data management plan in its proposal. Ideally, it needs to work equally well manually as well as digitally. The ethnographer normally does not have the time or energy to change data management procedures midethnography. Thus, the system needs to be ready before the ethnographer leaves home and should be robust enough to survive the fieldwork.

Also, both the journal and the interview notes should be stored separately. Database management is the first stage of analysis. The universality of language structure and logic makes vital the careful maintenance of what ethnographers hear and what they see. It is also indispensable for ethnographers to begin understanding and analyzing foreign cultural knowledge systems and to protect their analysis against bias. Not only do ethnographers manage recorded interviews and texts. They also structure interviews and document the steps they take to focus on the questions they use for follow-up.

Longer-term data storage is also necessary for analysis, both in the field and afterward. Ethnographers need to review the transcribed interviews while in the field in order to modify and enhance the interview questions. Initial data analysis can rely on a word search utility to conduct partial or preliminary indexing. Nowadays, these are available—in English, at least—on Adobe or Microsoft software. The researcher needs to create an index as soon as there is an interview in computer-readable form. Such an index should have integrity sufficient to organize data yet be flexible enough to be modified as more data arrive. After indexing, it is necessary to check the resulting word list. This consultation provides a more reliable method of appraising the content of interview texts. At that point, the only bottleneck is transcription.

If all else fails, digital transcription of interviews provides the opportunity not only for word searches but also for data mining. When attempting to elicit definitions, no single consultant will likely provide a complete definition of a term, with all the crucial attributes. Eliciting folk definitions is exceedingly important because it is a check on *semantic accent*—the ethnographer's tendency to define native terms with meanings that originate mostly in the culture of the ethnographer. As will be seen in Chapters 4 and 5, the folk definitions are analogous to an extensive bilingual dictionary that translates native terms into ordinary English explanations.

Any indexing program will do. One should be able to look at the index in two ways: in alphanumeric order and in order of word frequency.

The alphanumeric order is preferred by designers of indexing programs because it facilitates quick retrieval. Quick retrieval is particularly useful if the ethnographers know what they are looking for and are strongly committed to a theoretical orientation. An index by word frequency can make it easy to find out what an ethnographer *should* be looking for. Finally, it is necessary to be able to print the index. Software such as Adobe Acrobat is widely available and has at least some of the required capabilities.

Indexing software is generally not equipped to handle phrases very well. Some software will keep the words separated by dashes, so that key phrases can be hyphenated during transcription. This search method can be easy in languages the ethnographers know well, but it is impossible in languages over which they have no control.

Determining how sophisticated the data management system should be depends on the scale of the research. Ethnographic texts, journals, transcriptions, collected documents, and analytical structures are all collected in either actual or digital form in work papers. Werner, in his Hungarian fieldwork, set himself the goal of entering a minimum of 1,000 words, or 4 or at least 5 double-spaced typewritten pages, into his journal entries per day. In a year, that comes to about 365,000 words, or 1,460 pages.

On the other hand, I found that for 2-week rapid assessments, I might still record as many as 25 interviews. These interviews would last as long as an hour and a half. Two weeks was all I was given for each site visit in my work, so I had to rely on the hand-written steno-pad notes I took during the interviews as the platform from which to generate further questions and consider analysis. I, thus, could not analyze the interviews themselves until I left the field. With the notebook, I could at least keep track of the interviews. With the interview notes in front of me, I could devise follow-ups to elaborate on certain details.

Also, all the interviews were in English, which meant that I could use voice-activated software such as Dragon Naturally Speaking® for transcription. This convenience shortened the time taken for transcription. I could listen to an interview segment, mark the recorded segment's digital position in the transcription, and then recite what I had heard from the recorded interview segment.

The data management system is also governed by ethical issues of privacy and confidentiality. The two terms are often confused and need to be clarified. "Confidentiality" means that all information exchanged between the ethnographer and the consultant may be withheld from any third party. It refers to entire withholding of a name or other information from any third party. "Privacy" pertains more to control of access to personal and medical files and other similar files the disclosure of which would constitute a clearly unwarranted invasion of personal privacy.

THE PARTIES INVOLVED: PEER REVIEW AND INSTITUTIONAL REVIEW BOARDS

Depending on the nature of the written research proposal, the ethnographers may face a broad array of review organizations. This section will limit itself to scientific review, but we acknowledge that various humanities and philanthropic organizations have their own. The principal aim of the review system is for a proposal to undergo a quality control process in which the scientific merit of a product is critically reviewed and evaluated by independent peers. This book defines peers as persons who are not associated directly or indirectly with the product under review and whose background and expertise put them on par technically and scientifically with the authors of the product. We can categorize peers broadly as external and internal. Internal peer review is a review by individuals within the organization to which the ethnographer belongs. External peer review is an assessment by independent experts from outside the ethnographer's institutional organization. Blind review occurs when the identity of the reviewers is not made known to the authors.

Research proposals will all have to withstand review of varying intensity. There are three kinds of review that ethnographers encounter in the evaluation of proposals or review of reports. The first is the review by the ethnographer's academic professors or administrative supervisors within the organization or agency. These will not be discussed in this book in any great detail, other than to emphasize the importance of following whatever rules and regulations are acknowledged by other institutions.

The second kind of peer review is by scientific or program peers either as part of the proposal review or for article publication. Ideally, its goal is to highlight shortcomings in the document's theory or methods of data gathering or analysis, and mandate remedies. Such a review is usually binding. That is, failure to address the recommended remedies for noted shortcomings will usually result in denial of a project's funding or clearance for publication.

Institutional Review Boards

The third kind of review is to guarantee protection of human subjects in research. By law, protection of human participants is regulated under 45 C.F.R. 46, under the administration of the Department of Health and Human Services (DHHS):

> ... a systematic investigation, including research development, testing, and evaluation, designed to develop or *contribute to generalizable knowledge.* Activities that meet this definition constitute research for purposes of this policy, whether or not they are conducted or supported under a program that is considered research for other purposes. For example, some demonstration and service programs may include research activities. (*U.S. Code of Federal Regulations*, n.d., 45 C.F.R. 46.102(g); italics added)

The regulations then list six activities that are deemed not to be research, including mostly education-related programs. However, if these activities are considered research, including scientific research, then they involve a "human subject." Under the regulations, a "human subject" is a

> living individual about whom an investigator (whether professional or student) conducting research: (i) Obtains information or bio specimens through intervention or interaction with the individual, and uses, studies, or analyzes the information or bio specimens; or (ii) Obtains, uses, studies, analyzes, or generates identifiable private information or identifiable bio specimens. (*U.S. Code of Federal Regulations*, n.d., 45 C.F.R. 46.102(g))

(The term "human subjects" as defined in these regulations is the same as "human participants.") This book joins the AAA in recognizing this definition of "subject" as including consultants being interviewed or observed as part of ethnography.

The DHHS regulations similarly define an "intervention" to include both the physical procedures by which information or biospecimens are gathered and manipulations of the subject or the subject's environment that are performed for research purposes (*U.S. Code of Federal Regulations* 45 C.F.R. 46(e)(ii)). Even ethnographic interviews or observations can apply under this definition if the project is found to constitute research. Thus, a proposal writer is urged to read the *American Anthropological Association Statement on Ethnography and Institutional Review Boards* (AAA, 2004) and track its conclusions through a review of the definitions contained in 45 C.F.R. 46.

Sometimes ethnography has not been considered to be research because its findings are not considered "generalizable." For example, the U.S. Office of Management and Budget (OMB) decided that oral history conducted by the National Park Service did not require IRB review because

> oral history interviewing activities, in general, are not designed to contribute to generalizable knowledge and, therefore, do not involve research as defined by DHHS regulations at 45 CFR 46.102(d) and do not need to be reviewed by an institutional review board (IRB). (Carome & DHHS, 2003)

According to OMB (2002), "'influential,' when used in the phrase 'influential scientific, financial, or statistical information,' refers to disseminated information that OMB determines will have a clear and substantial impact on important public policies or important private sector decisions."

The AAA (2004) statement considers ethnography subject to IRB review, and it is therefore recommended that any ethnographer submitting a proposal review the AAA statement as well as refer to *U.S. Code of Federal Regulations* (n.d.), 45 C.F.R. 46.

Elements of Peer Review of Project and Proposal

The ethnographic process has always been a public one with many audiences. One audience is the native consultants and co-researchers. Others include the funding agencies and various academic and governmental peers. All will want to review some aspect of the research, and all may want to see who was interviewed. Ethnographers have attempted to guarantee confidentiality by not naming the individuals, giving them fictitious names, or withholding individual identities outright. The exemptions under the Freedom of Information Act (1967) allow at least some privacy but not confidentiality. Thus, inquiry directly undertaken or funded by the federal government involves introducing a prospective interviewee with what the Freedom of Information Act exemptions allow and do not allow. The question becomes when and when not to seek qualified legal advice.

Associated with privacy are also issues such as copyright and ownership of information. If the project is funded by the federal government of the United States, the information generated from it becomes part of the public domain. It cannot be withheld by the consultant unless agreed on in the contract. In short, privacy is important and increasingly difficult to observe. *Ethnographers should not promise consultants what cannot be delivered.* They need to obtain, moreover, the outline of a legal background on what they can and cannot do. This outline should be sufficient to encourage ethnographers to consult with legal experts before they get into trouble.

Ethnographic Sampling

A cognitive ethnographic proposal needs to contain a plan for how to select people for interview. While this planning begins before the research starts, it is crucial to understand that developing or negotiating a sampling process will continue into the fieldwork itself.

First, the ethnographer needs to obtain any information available on the target population's demographics, history, accessibility, government relations, and economy, and the required research permits. Moreover, agencies and other organizations with which ethnographers must deal in the field may have different ideas.

Second, ethnographers must be sure that the sampling procedure is representative. *A representative sample ensures that an ethnographer implements methods that obtain consultants the consensus of whose knowledge provides as complete a view of a social group's knowledge system as possible.* This definition means that ethnographers do not necessarily deal as much in the distribution of knowledge as in obtaining a consensus on what this knowledge comprises. These deceptively modest requirements presuppose that ethnographers can select people who know what they are talking about. Then, they must be able to determine whether the contradictions or differences in how the knowledge is obtained reflect incomplete research, the variability of a knowledge system found among individuals, differences that reflect the classes of people within a group, or differences that are indicative of different cultural outlooks.

These research questions make ethnographic sampling very different from probability, or statistical, sampling. Probability sampling depends on applying a design that ensures that everybody within a given population has an equal chance of being selected for the sample. This approach ensures that any kind of selective bias is avoided that would distort the distribution of knowledge throughout a population. Ethnographic sampling makes it possible to select people based on how much knowledge they have. Ethnographers want to characterize the *whole knowledge* of a people or group, not the *distribution* of some of its traits within that group.

Ethnographers thus have to take issues of sampling into account *before* entering the field, and to be prepared to negotiate and adapt research designs *throughout* the fieldwork. There are four major kinds of ethnographic sampling: (1) opportunistic sampling, (2) judgmental sampling, (3) ethnographic adaptations of probability sampling, and (4) face-to-face network sampling.

Opportunistic Sampling

Sometimes the selection of the research site is predetermined by factors external to the research design. For example, a governmental or other agency may have selected a group or class of people for research without the researcher's involvement, or there may be limitations of time and funding. In addition, someone will recommend a site because they have contacts there. If ethnographers have any say, they are best reminded of a very important rule of thumb: When confronted with the inevitable limitations of time, funding, interests of sponsorship, and accessibility, *it is best to concentrate on the group of people about whom the least is known.*

A good example comes from James Spradley's 1970 book *You Owe Yourself a Drunk*. He was asked to do an ethnography describing the interaction of homeless men, an alcohol rehabilitation program that was available to them, and the police. Spradley decided that he could not cover all three very well and selected the group about whom he knew the least—the homeless.

Another example is from the *Six Navajo School Ethnographies* (Werner et al., 1976). It shows in detail how the ethnographers developed a defensible sampling design by accounting for features within the social organization of Navajo schools during the mid-1970s. Here, it would have been optimal to study the interaction of school system administration, community, and student body.

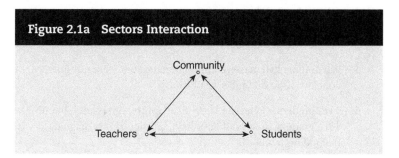

Figure 2.1a   Sectors Interaction

Community

Teachers   Students

Figure 2.1b   Sector Overlap

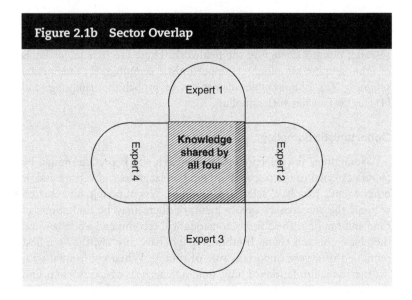

Due to insufficient time, the ethnographers decided to concentrate on the students—the least known segment of the triangle.

Once the ethnographers obtained tribal support for concentrating on the students, they had to acknowledge that they could not interview all the students in all of the six schools. They relied on their teaching experience to choose the most knowledgeable students among the different age-groups. Their experience had revealed that

1. 2nd-grade students seemed to know what the primary grades are all about but were not preoccupied with the 3rd or 4th grade;

2. 5th graders had learned what the elementary school system was about but, unlike 6th graders, had not begun to focus themselves on the next age-group;

3. 9th graders had mastered middle school but were not fully concentrating on high school; and

4. 11th graders had learned how to adapt to high school, but unlike 12th graders, they would not have set their sights on goals beyond high school.

Then, sampling shifted from opportunistic to network. At all grade levels, the ethnographers agreed that the classroom teachers would select the initial group of students to be interviewed. In addition to helping select articulate students to interview, consulting the teachers reduced their possible anxiety and helped secure their full cooperation. The researchers then tried to select the students who were mentioned in the interviews. These could include students who had problems or who were problems to others. See below for further discussion on network sampling.

Judgmental Sampling

Judgmental sampling is also known as purposeful, or purposive, sampling (Palinkas et al., 2013). In this design, individuals are selected according to certain criteria important to the ethnographer's research. The primary criterion is assessing individuals who are the most knowledgeable about the subject being studied.

Adaptations of Probability Sampling

Qualitative analogs to statistical sampling include random sampling and cluster sampling, among possible others. In normal random sampling, a researcher starts with a complete list, or census, of the people residing in an area. Each individual is assigned a number, and the researcher selects the individual by referring to a generator of random numbers. Werner and Bernard (1994) emphasize that a random sample

establishes what is typical in a social system. . . . In an ethnographic sample we usually have no idea what is typical. We work with key consultants, often experts, on topics like witchcraft, hunting, manioc planting, etc. Not knowing where to start, we start anywhere, often close to our entry point [to a cultural group]. We develop our network of contacts from there and the [result] is anything but random. (p. 8)

An example illustrates how a simulated random sample was applied for ethnography. A team of ethnographers conducted an ethnographic evaluation of a Navajo-controlled community school. They first obtained a list of parents who had had students enrolled at the school at one time or another. From this list, a 10% random sample was selected for interview (Platero et al., 1983).

Another probability sampling analog, known as area sampling, was comparable to the cluster sampling design (Cochran, 1977; Lang et al., 2004). Fanale (1982) first estimated the overall Navajo population. She then estimated density by (1) estimating that an area of 3 square miles contains, on average, three Navajo households. She then (2) divided her study area into a grid of 3 square-mile units, (3) sampled the squares randomly, and (4) censused, or selected all of, the households in the squares sampled.

Afterward, she conducted open-ended interviews of the residents on their livestock raising practices and obtained oral histories of the effects of the 1930s' federal Livestock Reduction on them.

Network Sampling

Network sampling is the most common form of sampling in ethnography. The approach starts with either an opportunistic or a judgmental sample. Then, the ethnographer asks each consultant to name other persons they would recommend for interview. The named individuals and their connections with the referring consultant are the start of a network. A network sample is sometimes referred to as a "snowball sample." This term suggests that the sample simply aggregates people during the research, with little attention paid to the method. A documented network approach is more systematic and methodical precisely because it *documents* the contacts. At the least, this documentation can reveal a record of how the ethnographer chose the consultants. Better yet, further study may reveal more about the group. For more information, see Chapter 4.

How Many Is Enough?

Once the questions of what, where, when, and who are considered, the next question is "how many?" It is here that ethnography differentiates itself very sharply from more conventional survey research. As mentioned above, probability sampling (Cochran, 1977) is designed to guarantee that any individual within a population has the same chance to be selected as any other such individual. If the purpose of the sample is to describe the distribution of traits, such as attitude, throughout a population, then this sampling approach helps avoid bias that might distort the true distribution. A random sample "establishes what is typical in a social system (population)" (Werner & Bernard, 1994, p. 8). It follows that in random sampling, or any of its derivatives, the more people or other elements selected, the better. Sample numbers of more than 100 are not unusual (see McCarty, 1994). However, adequacy of sample size becomes a matter of probability estimate. As McCarty (1994) summarized,

> When all is said and done, sample size is often determined by budget constraints rather than by formulas. If the formula calls for 3000 responses at $10 each, and there is only $20,000 in the budget, ethnographers lived with 2000 surveys. There is nothing wrong with this, so long as one is aware of the effect this may have on confidence and precision. (p. 5)

For ethnography, the aim is to describe a knowledge system as precisely and as thoroughly as possible, not to estimate the distribution of its parts throughout a population. As Werner and Bernard (1994, p. 8) stated, ethnographic sampling helps establish "the range of phenomena . . . not the proportion of traits within a population at large." In many instances, the ethnographer may have little idea of what this knowledge is, much less how it is distributed. Ethnographers know that they have succeeded in describing a cultural knowledge system if they have achieved *consensus* within their sample.

A.K. Romney and colleagues (1986) developed a mathematical model that ascertained the number of individuals who might be needed for consensus. They first administered a general knowledge test to a preselected group of university students. From this larger group, they generated a small sample of students, some of whom demonstrated high expertise in whatever the subject. They then selected others who did not have this expertise. From all these responses, they developed a table that showed that good results describing a body of knowledge can be generated from as few as four people *if they demonstrate a high degree of cultural consensus.*

> Are we really justified in using as few as a half dozen subjects with only a few items? We feel that the answer is yes for the following reasons: (1) we have a very tight theory whose assumptions are very stringent; (2) we are working with very high concordance codes where consensus is high; (3) we are only trying to find one "correct" answer for a question rather than, say, differentiating questions on a continuous scale of tendency to be "true" or "false." (p. 327)

In short, ethnographers need not be obsessed about relatively small selections of people. In fact, interests might often be better served by interviewing a few highly knowledgeable people intensively. An appropriate number of individuals have been selected when the ethnographer experiences *saturation*—keeps hearing the same body of knowledge over and over again. Werner and Bernard (1994, p. 8) have found that "when three or more consultants agree on a fact with any homogeneous social system it is time to move on to another group that views things somewhat differently" (see Romney et al., 1986).

Planning ethnography is a balance between time and resources. Writing a proposal and reviewing it from time to time will help keep the ethnographer focused on what needs to be done. By taking stock periodically, the ethnographer establishes what has been accomplished and what remains to be done. Also, planning an ethnography bleeds into the conduct of ethnography itself. It is always useful to look at what needs to be done in relation to the available time left for the project, and make practical changes to the ethnography as it proceeds.

CHAPTER 3

THE SEMANTIC UNITY OF THE ETHNOGRAPHIC INTERVIEW

An understanding of the lexical-semantic field theory will help make clear how to structure a cognitive ethnographic interview. Grand-tour and mini-tour questions are both structured semantically through the MTQ schema (*modification*, M; *taxonomy*, T; and *queuing*, Q) first mentioned in Chapter 1. Moreover, a consultant's answer to a mini-tour question may generate further mini-tour questions, sometimes converting a mini-tour into a grand-tour question.

When beginning a grand-tour question, it is not unusual to simply ask the consultant, "What is this?" "Tell me all about . . . " "What does this mean?" or "What has this experience meant to you?" Other questions could include "Tell me all about what you do at school" or "What kinds of people are there?" Queuing will be most familiar to many people because it becomes the start of almost any story. Answers to questions such as "Tell me what happened" are often sequential.

Moreover, no one is required to use the same semantic relationship in follow-up mini-tour questions as in the grand tour. A grand-tour question of sequence can be followed by mini-tours of taxonomy or of modification. When it is time to ask follow-up, or mini-tour, questions about an event, the answers include events that are part of other events. Thus, *the semantic relationships of the mini-tour question do not have to be based on the same relationship as that of the grand-tour answer.*

To understand this flexibility further, this book will first discuss the MTQ schema and the lexical-semantic field theory in more detail.

THE LEXICAL-SEMANTIC FIELD
THEORY AND THE MTQ SCHEMA

The lexical-semantic field theory is at the heart of cognitive ethnographic theory. The theory shows that terms take on meaning through their semantic relationships with other terms within the field. These relationships enable to understand an unknown term through a known term and communicate these terms to others. While the meaning of the terms may differ from one language to another, or in some cases do not exist, the semantic relationships among them do not vary. As discussed briefly in Chapter 1, Casagrande and Hale (1967) identified 13 different relationships common to all languages. From among these 13 relationships, Werner and Topper (1976) derived 3 relationships that could be used in turn to derive all the other 13: modification, taxonomy, and queuing. These three relationships are the *atomic* relationships. No other kind of semantic relationship comprises or stands for them.

The MTQ schema show how the names of terms, and the semantic relationships among them, can be represented in a unified and coherent whole, or field.

Taxonomy and Taxonomic Trees

Having somebody name all the kinds of things that are denoted by a term is an *extensional* definition. It is a great start, but it can become cumbersome. The *intensional* definition is a better way to identify attributes that show information about that term. An intensional definition tells someone how to determine what is or is not denoted by a given term. A good definition usually relies on a combination of intensional and extensional attributes.

Thus, it is imperative to figure out a way of getting a manageable set of attributes that show what X are a kind of Y and what are not. The following statements accomplish answering this question of what is or is not:

- B is an A (or B is a kind of A).

- All B are A, but not all A are B. (This relation is set theoretical and not semantic.)

It is possible to diagram the relationship between A and B:

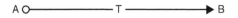

A O————————— T —————————▶ B

Here, A and B are labels for the nodes, which are related to each other through taxonomy, or T. The statements "B is a kind of A" and "*not* A is a kind of B" are both true. This asymmetric relationship explains the arrow from A to B.

A taxonomic relationship means "All B are A, and *not* all A are B." If we then add the term "C" such that "C is a kind of A," then "C *contrasts* with B" and "B *contrasts* with C." The tree diagram appears in Figure 3.1. The nodes are labeled as A, B, and C. The arrows are labeled by the taxonomic relation, T.

In Figure 3.1, the statements "B is a kind of A" and "C is a kind of A" are true but *not* "B and C are kinds of each other." Thus, B and C are in *contrast* to each other in some way, as kinds of A. A tree diagram makes the taxonomic levels of classification easier to follow.

Modification (Attribution) and Folk Definitions

Attribution modifies a term, or referent, by providing other terms and phrases that tell the listener more about the word's meaning. Modifiers can appear in the form of simple sentences, phrases, or even another single term. The referent, plus its accompanying phrases, constitutes a *folk definition*. To understand how taxonomy works, it is best to include a discussion of the folk definition.

A word of caution is necessary. Dictionary definitions are constructed around a term and its attributes, but the definition is often condensed so that the semantic relationships are not always obvious. The definition of the English word "stone" illustrates this. In folk definitions, the attributes are fully articulated as discrete sentences or phrases. Definitions such as those found in a dictionary are often highly abbreviated and somewhat difficult to follow. An example of a formal definition of a "stone" is the one in *Merriam-Webster Dictionary*.

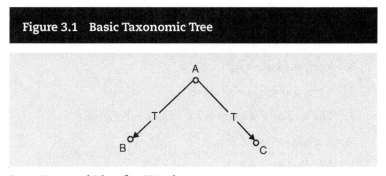

Figure 3.1   Basic Taxonomic Tree

Source: Werner and Schoepfle, 1987, vol 1.

Dictionary Definition: "Stone"

1. a concretion of earthy or mineral matter: concretion of indeterminate size or shape; [such as] rock is a kind of stone; a piece of rock for a specified function: such as a building block, a paving block, a precious stone [or] gem, gravestone, grindstone, whetstone, as more of a surface upon which a drawing, text, or design to be lithographed is drawn or transferred

2. something resembling a small stone: such as . . . calculus, the hard central portion of a drupaceous fruit (such as a peach), a hard stony seed (as of a date)

3. . . . any of various units of weight; especially . . . an official British unit equal to 14 pounds

4. curling stone, round playing piece used in various games

5. a stand or table with a smooth flat top on which to impose or set type.

Converting this to a folk definition involves breaking it down into its basic sentence or phrase attributes, to make the dictionary definition more like a folk definition constructed in ethnography.

Folk Definition of a Stone

1. A stone is a [kind of] concretion of earthly mineral matter.

2. A stone is a kind of mineral.

3. A stone is like a rock.

4. A paving block is a kind of stone.

5. A whetstone is a kind of stone.

6. A gem is a kind of stone.

7. A gravestone is kind of stone.

8. The hard core of a seed in a fruit is a kind of stone.

9. A stone is a kind of weight.

10. A curling stone is a kind of stone.

11. A stand or table with a smooth flat top on which to impose or set type is a kind of stone.

12. A stone has indeterminate size or shape.

Attributes 2 to 12 are taxonomic but do not modify directly. We are left with "a stone is a concretion of earthly mineral matter that has indeterminate size or shape." The problem with the dictionary definition is that a stone can belong to multiple taxonomies. Thus, the definition would have to refer to stones as minerals, tools, adornments, furniture, or plants. A conventional dictionary, at best, contains an overview of references to a broad domain of meaning.

The following example of a folk definition comes from *Six Navajo School Ethnographies* (Werner et al., 1976). Young Navajo students describe kinds of teachers. Note that in many of these Navajo definitions, the consultant is bilingual and blends English and Navajo in his or her description. At times, in fact, the student will redundantly describe a teacher in both languages. Navajo comments are thus included here because speakers occasionally code-switched Navajo and English when they were talking.

Definition of a Very Good Teacher

1. *Ayógo bił bééhózin* (The teacher really knows what she is doing).

2. The teacher gets mad only when we are naughty.

3. *Łahda éí ashiiké be'édadíláahgo yich'a hashkée łeh* (Sometimes when the boys are naughty, the teacher gets after them).

4. *Háká'análwo' łeh* (The teacher helps us).

5. *Chééh ájił'įigo 'kónáánát'é' hałníigo* (If you can't do something, he tells us, "This is the way to do this").

6. *Doo t'óó báhádzidgo yíhoniłka'daákonidi tsįį łgo ni'dzizogo t'éíyá* (He doesn't force us, but you have to be writing fast).

7. *Díí tsįįłgo ádadoołííł nihiłnii łeh; ałdó' ákonidi bídaadoołaahgo índaǫsignout nihiłniiłłeh* (Teacher tells us, "Do these in a hurry, but learn them, then sign out").

8. *'T'áadoo ahééda'oł'íní nihiłnii łeh* (The teacher tell[s] us, "Don't copy from another").

9. *Bił hózhǫǫ łeh* (The teacher is usually happy).

Figure 3.2 Navajo Classification and Definitions of Teachers

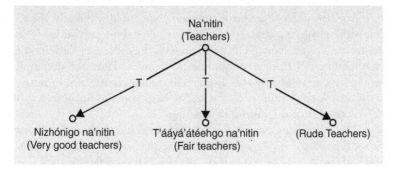

10. *Ayóogo yíneedlį̨́ na'natin łeh* (Teacher is interested in teaching).

11. *Áádóó t'áadoo'ádaoht'íní aají tsį́łgo da'íínólhta' nílę́į́ tsį̨́įłgo oolkił yiłniigo* (She tells them, "Don't do that; time is going fast; you better read and study over there").

12. *T'áá dinékehjí dóó t'áá bilagą́anaak'ehjí yína'niltin* ([Teacher] tells them in Navajo and English).

13. They go on field trips.

A good teacher, to Navajo elementary school students, is a kind of teacher.

This definition is an element of a taxonomic classification, as illustrated in a tree diagram of Navajo teachers (see Figure 3.2).

Note that the consultant, a Navajo elementary school student, emphasizes qualities of interpersonal compatibility with the teachers as well as their ability to teach. These definitions became more important as the ethnographic analysis proceeds, since they help researchers derive hypotheses on how the young people valued their teachers, depending on interpersonal compatibility and teaching skills.

The following are the definitions of fair and rude teachers.

Definition of a Fair Teacher (*T'áá yá'átéehgo na'nitin*)

1. *Doo hashkéeda* (Does not get after us).

2. *Doo t'óó báhádzidgo* (Doesn't force us).

3. *Éiyá kónáádoohníí̜* (Tells us what to do).

4. *Teacherǫ́ígíí éiyáǫjó t'áadoole'é bijiníígó doo ayóogo át'ii̜da łeh ałdoó'* (When you ask [the teacher] for something he hardly does it).

Definition of Rude Teachers

5. *T'áádoole'é saad t'áá ákó'jiił'íi̜hgo doo ákó'iinilaada' hałniih hane'dǫ́ę́' nínéidiił ts'i̜ilh łeh* (The sentences will be right, he says, "You made it wrong," and then hits you on the back).

6. *Rubberbandǫda ałch'i̜' yee adilą́sh łeh* (He shoots rubber bands at another teacher).

7. *Ałdó' timeǫkóníłtsoh dahnaazhilígíí éí ałdó' doohah'oolkiłgóó t'óó díigi' át'ée náás yidiłhki'. Kodi doohah yi̜níshta'góó, índa daats'i twoǫpage honisdziihgo t'óó ch'i̜néijah, éí biniinaa ałdó'* (Also, there is a big time clock—one that hangs [from the wall]—he moves the hands forward, even when I still have about two pages to go. We go out anyway. That's why he's rude too).

These definitions of good, fair, and rude teachers came from transcriptions of interviews of students from only one school. To the researcher, the definitions appear oriented toward evaluating both the interpersonal rapport with the teacher and his or her ability. These impressions of the researcher became the source of hypotheses that could be tested later.

The following definition shows how the folk definition can help structure a description in an English interview. This interview is with a National Park Service employee about his experiences during the September 11, 2001, terrorist bombings of the New York World Trade Center. The setting was Liberty Island, the location of the Statue of Liberty, where boatloads of New Yorkers were being ferried out of New York City so that they could be treated, triaged, or otherwise assisted. The National Park Service employees provided many of these services as the refugees arrived on Liberty Island.

Consultant: I mean, the first images of what those people looked like were nothing like what one would've seen on TV later on in the days that followed that incident.

Ethnographer: How so?

Consultant: They literally—many people looked like they were in shock. People arriving on the island, many of them in business attire—both men, women, children, people with their pets. You could see that all of them were displaced in a very, very quick amount of time. No one had time to think. They just had to leave and escape. And . . .

And they looked like living ghosts. They were completely covered in debris, dust. People were injured. Some of them didn't even know that they were injured. Some of them didn't care that they were injured. They just wanted to leave. And I guess not having seen what they were seeing or they had seen while they were trying to leave, we were then seeing the real magnitude of what was going on in the city and that this was only a brief taste of the horror that everyone was going through in downtown New York.

There were several hundred people who were placed on boats who—some of them were decontaminated with hoses to just allow them to be able to breathe—a lot of them with respiratory symptoms.

Again, the first step is to summarize in outline form how the consultant saw the people who had been ferried to Liberty Island.

[People were ferried to Liberty Island who were] nothing like what we would've seen on TV.

1. "*All* were displaced in a very, very quick amount of time."
   a. No one had time to think.
   b. They just had to leave and escape.
   c. [Many arrived] in business attire—both men, women, children, people with their pets.
   d. Many looked like they were in shock.

2. "*Many* people [of them] looked like they were in shock."
   a. Many were injured.
   b. They didn't even know they were injured.
   c. They just wanted to leave.
   d. Some didn't care that they were injured.

3. "*Some* looked like living ghosts."

   a. They were completely covered in debris, dust.

   b. Some of them were decontaminated with hoses to just allow them to be able to breathe.

   c. A lot of them with respiratory symptoms.

By focusing on what the consultant meant by "nothing like what we would've seen on TV," three definitions immediately emerge from his description.

Definition: People Displaced in a Very, Very Quick Amount of Time

1. No one had time to think.

2. They just had to leave and escape.

3. They arrived in business attire—both men, women, children, people with their pets.

Definition: People Who Looked Like They Were in Shock

1. Many were injured.

2. They didn't even know they were injured.

3. They just wanted to leave.

4. Some didn't care that they were injured.

Definition: People Who Looked Like Living Ghosts

1. They were completely covered in debris, dust.

2. Some of them were decontaminated with hoses to just allow them to be able to breathe.

3. A lot of them with respiratory symptoms.

By focusing on the definitions and their attributes, a tree diagram can show how the consultant's description is semantically structured. The basic relationship of modification can be shown as

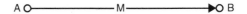

A O———————— M————————▶O B

Figure 3.3   Definition of People Ferried to Liberty Island

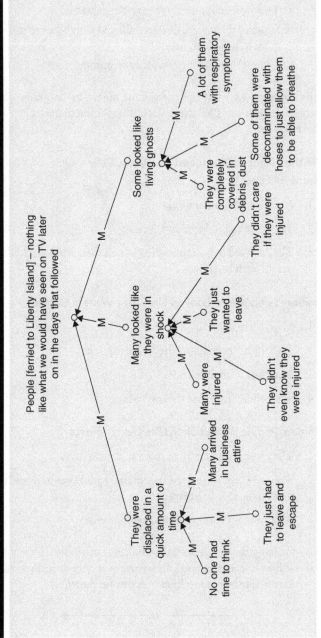

Source: Author created based on data from United States Government Department of the Interior, National Park Service. 2004, Policies for Managing Cultural Resources.

or read as "A modifies B." This basic relationship can then be applied to the tree diagram in Figure 3.3. While its present form provides little additional information, the interview might generate a second level of attributes. It is clear that even a simple folk definition can help structure descriptions of conditions in an interview.

An interview with more than one person requires close attention not only to how individual speakers overlap and disagree with one another. The following example is part of a study conducted in San Juan County, New Mexico (Tonigan, 1982). The study evaluated a proposal to combine two predominantly Navajo Indian school districts and form them into a single district that would be distinct from the rest of the county. The two districts were Shiprock, located on the Navajo reservation, and Kirtland, located off the reservation. As part of this evaluation, a team of ethnographers interviewed Navajo students from both districts who would be grouped together into the proposed new district. While both sets of students were predominantly Navajo, the Navajos in Kirtland District were considered more acculturated than those in Shiprock District. The simple question was how the Navajos in either district viewed the situation. The answers show that the students had negative views of each other. We are indebted to Rose T. Morgan for conducting these interviews and setting up the definitions.

The first definition is from the standpoint of the Kirtland students toward those in Shiprock. The Navajo-speaking Shiprock students appeared to go out of their way to make the Kirtland students feel ill at ease. The Kirtland students described the Shiprock students in this way.

Definition: Shiprock Students

1. They are hard to get along with.

2. They live in the old ways.

3. They eat traditional foods.

4. They speak Navajo, and many of us don't.

5. They are not nice to me.

6. They would say things in Navajo and give me funny looks.

7. I don't speak Navajo, and I don't see why they have to act that way.

8. They drink down there.

9. They get more homework there than they do here, but the students [there] fight a lot.

10. They even fight with teachers.

The second definition is from the viewpoint of Shiprock students. It highlights the differences between the two groups of Navajos.

Definition: Kirtland Students

1. I wouldn't be their friend if they were the last people on earth.

2. Anybody [that] goes to Kirtland is no friend of mine.

3. They call us Johns.

4. They feel that the kind of school and the kind of courses they have are better than the ones in Shiprock.

5. They say we are no good, that students here like to smoke and drink all the time.

Although there are only 5 attributes from the Shiprock students and 10 from the Kirtland students, the Shiprock definition is not more simply constructed. The public schools in the *Six Navajo School Ethnographies* (Werner et al., 1976) helped explain how "Johns" were students who (1) lived in the rural areas of the reservation, (2) lived in traditional hogans, (3) ate traditional foods such as mutton stew and fried bread, and (4) spoke predominantly Navajo and spoke English with a pronounced Navajo accent. As a result of these markers, they were often considered less intelligent and less knowledgeable about the urban life that was part of a normal public school student's daily life. The Shiprock students saw themselves as more "John" because they still had more ties with life on the Navajo reservation. Thus, the term when used by a Kirtland student carried a pejorative weight to it.

In the next example, the researchers constructed a taxonomy from the definitions of attitudes toward mining development on Navajo land. It relies on another Navajo study, about a community of individuals who were faced with a proposed strip mine that was to extend through the middle of their community. Here, the ethnographers interviewed the consultants about their personal experiences in dealing with the coal companies, the Bureau of Indian Affairs, the Navajo tribal government, and one another. Describing their own experiences, they compared themselves with others within their community. These conversations

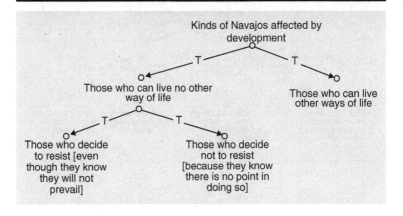

Figure 3.4   Kinds of Navajos Affected by Energy Development

Kinds of Navajos affected by development

Those who can live no other way of life

Those who can live other ways of life

Those who decide to resist [even though they know they will not prevail]

Those who decide not to resist [because they know there is no point in doing so]

were mostly in Navajo, and the ethnographers wanted to see if they could establish an overall classification of people that represented some consensus within the community. The initial taxonomic tree diagram proposed by Kenneth Begishe and Rose Morgan described the kinds of individuals according to the options they would choose should development occur (see Figure 3.4).

The tree indicates that the Navajos of this community affected by development divided themselves into two classes: (1) those who can live no other life and (2) those who can live other ways of life. Of the former, there are those who resist, even if they know it is fruitless, and those who do not resist, precisely because they consider it futile.

Begishe and Morgan prepared the taxonomic diagram, which was written in Navajo, and then narrated it at a community meeting. The Navajos indicated no difficulty following this information, and one of the individuals, seen as a leader among the group, commented in Navajo (Schoepfle et al., 1979),

> Me too, I like this—that this, the way this research has been presented. You see, when things are researched in depth, then it is clear that the kinds of people you describe do indeed emerge. There are indeed those who want change, those who say "no" and the group that says "wait a minute, easy!" whose members are here at this meeting tonight. . . . In this way I believe and

Figure 3.5 Kinds of Navajo

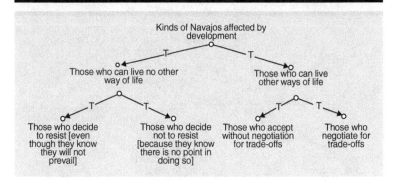

hope that things will change for the better. Right now we do not understand one another and that is the reason for the present [factionalism and confusing conditions]. (p. 84)

To the ethnographers, this comment appeared as a very gracious and polite criticism. From this quote, we realized that an entire category of individuals had been omitted—those who could live other ways of life but were willing to negotiate for better conditions on behalf of those who could not. The research team modified the taxonomic tree as shown in Figure 3.5.

The Navajos provided definitions for each one of these "Kinds of Navajos Affected by Development" in Navajo, the language with which everyone was the most at ease in speaking. Thus, the definition for those willing to negotiate for mitigations was "They say, 'Easy, let's find out more about the other'."

Definition: Those [Navajos] Who Negotiate for Mitigations

1. They say, "Easy, easy, let's find out more about the other."
   (*Hazhó'ó **hazhó'ó** bééhózinígo t'áá át'é*)

2. They are the group that says, "Wait a minute; take it easy."

3. They wish things would change for the better.

4. "I stand firmly by saying that I will not give up my sheep permit" [these people say].

5. In the near future, we will have to accept this very situation (i.e., of having to move away from this area) [they say].

6. "The white man still do [does] not understand our view" [they say].

The following definition, "We do not come to understand one another" provides more insight into "Let's find out more about the other."

Definition: Those Navajos Who Can Live No Other Way of Life

1. We do not come to understand one another.

2. We throw words at each other.

3. It is true that for lack of knowledge of others we are unkind to one another.

The consultants hoped that by seeing all of the different attitudes displayed together logically, the diagram itself might become a means of planning. For the ethnographers, moreover, this critique and the changes to the tree diagram forced them to focus more on a systematic approach to understanding the kinds of mitigations, or trade-offs, the Navajos in this community would like to see. Chapter 5 will show how the research team focused on the effects of forced resettlement involved with both mining and agribusiness development. The discussion will show how a decision model for mitigations was proposed and tested on a wider population of Navajos.

Queuing

The third atomic relationship is queuing or sequence. It states that for two referents A and B, one occurs or is perceived before another. It follows that for B and C, the same kind of relationship applies. The overall relationship is best expressed in this diagram:

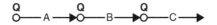

The arrows denote the referents A, B, and C. The nodes represent queuing, or "and then." The diagram reads as "A, and then B, and then C." This relationship makes no statement about time, duration, or

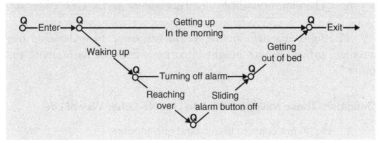

Figure 3.6 Getting Up in the Morning

Source: Adapted from Werner and Schoepfle (1987b).

whether A is a precondition for B or B for C. All that queuing means is that one thing occurs or is perceived before or after another.

Queuing brings up the complex logical and semantic relationship of *part–whole* as well, in addition to the MTQ relationships. Here, an activity or an event will include events that make up its parts. The diagram of weekday getting up in the morning (see Figure 3.6) demonstrates this.

The diagram also shows that *verbal action plans* (VAPs) are hierarchical and the semantic relationship part–whole for waking up is a part of getting up in the morning. Similarly included are turning off the alarm and getting out of bed. When this sequence of activities is conducted as a routine, it is known as a *plan*, or VAP.

SPECIALIZED MTQ INTERVIEW TECHNIQUES

Other interview questions can be analyzed through the MTQ schema but do not fall into the categories discussed already. Three of these are debriefing, slip sorting, and word association. There are doubtless others that a researcher can generate.

Debriefing

The term *debrief* was developed in the military as a meeting and process to review formally what happened on a mission. Subsequently, it has acquired various specialized meanings in business. The *Webster Dictionary* definition for the transitive verb "debrief" is "to interrogate [someone]" in order to obtain useful information. The dictionary's secondary definition is "to carefully review upon completion," a preferable definition despite its lack of detail. The primary reason for preferring the second one is ethical. Ethnographic debriefing does not involve interrogation. The most familiar form of interrogation, the Reid technique, is used primarily by law enforcement officials and involves processes (Hirsch, 2014; Inbau et al., 2015; Orlando, 2014) that are beyond the scope of ethnography.

Ethnographic debriefing proceeds in four phases (Schoepfle & Werner, 1999): (1) preparation, (2) debriefing for content, (3) debriefing for context, and (4) debriefing for quantification. *Preparation* for a debriefing bears two ground rules. The first is egalitarianism. That is, everyone is there for one purpose: to coproduce an accurate description. It is not intended to highlight the knowledge or memory of one participant at the expense of another's. It also means that all participants must be equally open to being corrected. Finally, it means that everyone agrees to one major rule: *If you don't know, you don't know.*

Thus, if somebody cannot answer a question, it does not reflect adversely on his or her ability, or even performance. It simply means that the individual does not have the information to answer the question. If someone feels threatened by some kind of adverse evaluation, they will reasonably become defensive. This defensiveness will interfere with learning or even tempt the speaker to invent something. Ethnographic debriefing, thus, is a form of nonthreatening instruction.

The second ground rule is orderliness. In corporate or business settings, there are often plans and rules for debriefings. Here, the goal is to conduct a form of group interview. One person takes the lead to ensure that the interview remains systematic and focused on the topic. It also means that this person enforces the nonevaluative egalitarianism on which all participants should agree.

Debriefing for content, the second phase, is the heart of the debriefing process. The strategy and logic are the same as in conducting grand-tour and mini-tour interviews, and are structured around the MTQ schema. Ethnographic debriefing can thus start out as an interview about a participant's interview, observation, experience, or report.

Debriefing for context, the third phase, involves the same reasoning and strategy as in Phase 2, but it differs in its focus. It focuses on the *context* of the event being recounted, or "the events that surround the main event, the elicited knowledge or other content elicited in Phase 2" (Schoepfle & Werner 1999, p. 161). For example, if someone has provided a summary of a major meeting, the interviewer may wish to elicit information about the sequence of specific events. Interviews about sequence or queuing are the best method to make the information systematic. The interviewers may ask for every conceivable detail that happened at this meeting regardless of how unimportant the event may have appeared to the one recounting the event. This might involve part–whole, taxonomy, or any other semantic relation.

Debriefing for quantification, the fourth phase, requires eliciting information on counting, measurement, exact time or date of occurrence, and immediate antecedents or consequents. Many times, the person debriefed may not have been able to pay adequate attention to such detail but may be able to bracket answers to these questions. With bracketing, the speaker provides information on events that occurred before, during, or after the event in question, for which they may know the date or time. For example, the person being debriefed may be able to bracket when a family reunion occurred by recalling important events that occurred before or after it. Or a reporter may estimate the number of people attending an event by recalling the size of the room, camp, or house in which the event occurred. In other situations, a speaker can estimate the number of guests at a ceremony by being able to recall the number of sheep brought for feeding them.

Slip Sorting

The following interview involved a high school student, S, who was discussing the different kinds of students encountered in his school; E stands for the ethnographer.

Student Interview

E: **When** you go to classes throughout the day, I guess you encounter different kinds of students. Rather than my asking you what kinds of students there are, could I have you take any class you have throughout the day—it doesn't matter what class—and just list the people in that class, one name to a card? And then group these cards any way you want?

S: **Like** how?

E: **Anywhere** you want.

S: **Okay.** [Both pause] Right now?

E: **Sure,** take your time. . . . And when you have the names on these cards, put the cards in different stacks, any way you want, according to any rule you like. [Both pause.]

S: Okay. [The student writes down the names of the other students on the cards and places them in different stacks.]

E: Okay, I see five different piles of cards here; how are they different?

S: By their ability in class.

E: Uh-huh.

S: Well, [first file] Darlene, Doris, and Brian—they understand it pretty good—they can get it to their head and keep it there. And [second pile] Geraldine, Jennifer, Betty, and Phil—they're all about the same. I guess they understand it too and keep it in their head, but they disagree about some things they have to do.

E: Uh-huh.

S: Then, [third pile] Kim and Jerry—they just take the notes down. I guess they remember it.

E: They take the notes down and memorize them, you say?

S: So they remember it, I guess.

E: I see, and the next group?

S: Kathy and Beverly, Bobby and Phyllis [fourth pile]—they just fool around in that class; they get it a few times, not really all the time. And Gloria and Betty [fifth pile]—they just don't care, I guess.

E: Don't care?

S: They don't learn anything in there.

E: When you mention the first group and the second group, you say they could keep it in their head, but the second group disagree with what they have to do?

S: Yeah.

E: I'm not clear.

S: Well, they can get it, they can remember, they don't really forget.

E: Don't care as long as they get a good grade?

S: Yeah, just so they learn it; something like that.

E: And in the second group, they can keep it in their head, but they disagree on what they have to do.

S: **Yeah,** they say they like what they're being taught or don't like what they are being taught.

E: **When** you say they don't agree with what is being taught, what are some of the ways in which they don't agree—like, what did they say?

S: **How** the teacher teaches it, what kind of assignments he gives—I think that's it.

E: **Okay,** in the third group, they take down notes and memorize?

S: **Well** I don't know if they memorize it, but they just take notes. I don't know if they learn anything or not.

E: **Do** they disagree with what's being taught? Do they ever disagree with the teacher?

S: **Not** really.

E: **I** see, and how do they differ, say, from those that don't care as long as they get a good grade?

S: **I** don't know [laughs].

E: **Okay,** the next group fools around and gets it a few times?

S: **Yeah,** well, they listen once in a while . . .

E: **Uh-huh.**

S: . . . to some stories that are, you know, some interesting stuff that they are being taught.

E: **And** how are they different, say, from those that disagree?

S: **Well,** they just never really listen . . . to what's being taught.

E: **Never** listen . . . ?

S: **Yeah,** just talking to each other all the time; they listen every once in a while.

E: **And** the fifth group—they don't care, and they learn nothing?

S: **Yeah,** they hardly come to class, and when the tests come, they just start saying stuff like they don't know what it's all about. The teacher tries telling them that they weren't here a certain time, when they were taught, but they don't—well, they just put anything on the test.

Going through the interview we get the following definitions and classifications:

Pile 1: Students who can get it through their head
- They understand it.
- They can keep it in their heads.

Pile 2: Students who can get it through their head
- They understand it.
- They can keep it in their heads.
- They disagree about some things they have to do.

Note that the titles were adjusted so that both piles could be contrasted the same way. At this point, Pile 2 looks like a subpile of Pile 1. Piles 3, 4, and 5 are labeled as follows:

Pile 3: Students who take down notes and memorize them
- Thus, they remember it.

Pile 4: Students who fool around in class
- They get it a few times, not really all the time.

Pile 5: Students who don't care
- They don't learn anything.

At this point, the ethnographer decided to probe further to see if there is some structure to the classification. The new attributes are listed as the consultant mentioned them for each group.

Pile 1
- They can get it.
- They can remember.
- They don't really forget.
- They don't really care what it is as long as they get a good grade.
- They just learn it.

Pile 2 (Just two attributes make Pile 2 different from Pile 1.)
- They say they like what they are being taught.
    or
- They say they don't like what they're being taught.

Pile 3

- They take notes.
- They can remember it [see previous response].
- They may learn something.
- They don't disagree with what is being taught.

Pile 4

- They listen every once in a while to some stories.
- They listen to interesting stuff that they are being taught.
- They rarely listen.
- They just talk to each other all the time.

Pile 5

- They hardly come to class.
- When tests come, they say they don't know what it's all about; they just put anything on a test.

With all the attributes combined, three groups of students appear: (1) those who can "get it to their heads," (2) "students who will learn just anything" for a good grade, and (3) students who dislike some subjects and say so. Thus, the slip sorting, combined with further interviewing, results in the taxonomy shown in Figure 3.7.

This taxonomic tree diagram illustrates how the students "who can get it into their heads," "who take notes," "who fool around," and "who

Figure 3.7 Taxonomic Tree Derived From the Slip Sort: Kinds of Students

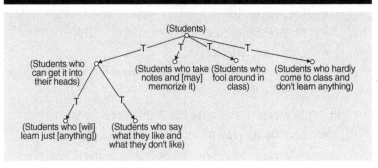

Source: Werner and Schoepfle 1987, vol 2.

hardly come to class" contrast with one another. The students who will learn just anything and those who say what they like and what they do not like, in turn, are kinds of students who can "get it into their heads" but contrast with one another.

Word Association Chains

Word association chains can be used to construct folk definitions by generating attributes for the term to be defined. The intent of the word association exercise is to generate a model of semantic knowledge, not to elicit terms that may reveal psychodynamic processes or attributes of personality. The consultant is asked to list as many words as he or she can associate with the referent term. The number of words someone can recall is usually around 5 ± 2. Then, the ethnographer asks the consultant to describe, usually in a single sentence or phrase, how the associated word is important to understanding the referent. These descriptions become the attributes of a folk definition.

The approach is particularly useful when consultants are reticent about volunteering attribute phrases. The reasons for the reticence are legion. Consultants may be shy about providing a definition for a term or talking about the meaning of the term in group situations. Or they may be children who are not yet accustomed to producing ordinary folk definitions with ease. Or, in some group situations, the consultant may be perfectly able to define the term but may be reluctant to venture a definition because they think the answer is obvious and they are being asked a "trick question." In other instances, the term for which the ethnographer is requesting a definition may be so abstract that they have difficulty generating attributes. Whatever the reason, rather than change the question or end the interview, the ethnographer can resort to an ethnographic word association.

Once the consultant has provided the terms and told the ethnographer how they consider them significant, the ethnographer can then present the answers back to the consultant and ask them what they think of the definition. Table 3.1 illustrates how a word can generate folk definitions. The consultant is asked to volunteer about five terms that come to mind when defining the English word "sincerity."

In this example, the consultant first mentions the terms "good person," "Honest Abe," and "bicentennial." The ethnographer then begins constructing the folk definition from the terms "honest" and "good person." The ethnographer generates the attributes "is a kind of honesty" and "is an attribute of a good person." Often, there is a "tail" in the

Table 3.1   Example of Word Association–Derived Definition

Examples of Word Association		Folk Definition From Word Association	
Stimulus word	Sincerity	Sincerity	• Is a characteristic of a good person • Is a kind of honesty
Response chain	Good person Honest Abe Bicentennial	Or	
Sincerity		Sincerity	• Is a kind of honesty • Is an attribute of a good person

Source: Werner and Schoepfle, 1987, vol 1.

chain. The "tail" contains attributes that provide no direct connection to the term "sincerity." Here, the tail includes terms such as "Honest Abe" and "bicentennial." The consultant associated these phrases with the term "sincerity" for whatever reason.

THE NATURAL HISTORY OF THE ETHNOGRAPHIC INTERVIEW

Chapter 3 discussed the basic or atomic semantic relationships that structure both how an interview is conducted and how it is analyzed afterward. These include *modification*, *taxonomy*, and *queuing*. These relationships are "atomic" because not only do they govern the conduct and analysis of the interview, they are also the basis of the theory that underlies cognitive ethnography. Chapter 4 will shift to the natural history of the interview itself. It describes the events within an interview that happen no matter what the kind of interview.

THE NATURAL HISTORY OF THE INTERVIEW

Figure 4.1 illustrates the natural history of a global interview plan, portrayed as sequence and part–whole. Notice that this diagram is a slightly more complex version of the plan for getting up in the morning

Figure 4.1   Plan and Subplans of an Interview

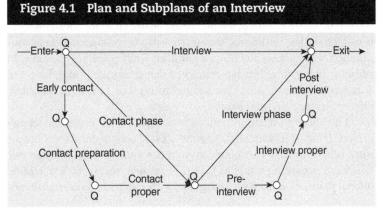

Source: Werner and Schoepfle (1987a).

in Chapter 3 (Figure 3.6). The diagram's arrows illustrate a *contact phase*, then the *interview proper*, and finally the *exit*.

The nodes where the arrows meet can be verbalized as "and then." Those activities that occur before and after the actual interview takes place are important to the success of the interview. While they appear to be a small part of the total interview process, they often take the greatest amount of time.

Contact Phase

Within the contact phase, there are early contact, contact preparation, and the contact itself. Early contact is made with the consultants for the purpose of setting up or scheduling the interview. As a general rule, people may be happy to talk to a person, but they may want time to think about what they are going to say. Even governmental or corporate officials need advance notification—at least a telephone call to arrange an interview time. For these corporate settings, the reader might review various books on job hunting and interviewing as further illustration. These books detail how repeated calls to the decision maker's office may be necessary (Bolles, 2018). Finally, when "studying up," it may be necessary to arrange through contacts to talk to the decision maker. If these arrangements are not made, one may find oneself talking to a public relations official, who will provide relatively little information (Ho, 2009).

When scheduling an interview with the Navajo Indians, on the other hand, Werner and his coworkers generally specified 4 days. In the southwestern United States, Native Americans attribute special properties to the number four, so it appealed to both the consultants as well as the ethnographer. It was also easy to remember. In Navajo culture, men often would check with their wives before they would consent to an interview. There is a solid, legend-based justification for such consultation. Even in less traditional settings, a 4-day waiting period made consultation with spouses and other significant family members possible. In addition, many older Navajos remarked that they were glad to have had 4 days to think over what they wanted to say. For further background, see "turn taking" in this chapter.

The contact preparation phase is common to all interviews in any project. It may start with a list of names, a list of geographical locations, or some other means of choosing consultants within a research design (see Chapter 2 regarding sampling). This phase may also include obtaining official permission from various agencies to contact certain consultants.

Such consultation is increasingly important because bureaucracies are indispensable to many applied research projects (Heyman, 2004). In addition to checking equipment, this phase is also a time to figure out how to identify other people to contact. For example, is there someone willing to make the introduction, take the ethnographer to the location of the consultants, explain the location of the consultant to the ethnographer, or bring the consultant to the ethnographer for the interview? Ultimately, how a contact is made will depend on the field situation, the affected agencies, and the location of the interview. It is for this reason that the ethnographer takes the time to review and compare the feasibility of the grass hut, muddy field, white room, and commuter research scenarios outlined in Chapter 2.

The contact proper allows all those involved to make introductions, explore possible relationships, explain the project or purpose of the interview, negotiate role relationships, and determine compensation, if any. Other issues may pertain to privacy, enlistment of relatives, ownership of interview recordings and transcripts, and additional people whom the researcher might interview. This contact phase may extend beyond the beginning of the interview itself. For example, in a research conducted at Rock Point School, the ethnographers found that they had to set up a randomized ethnographic sampling design. This design became necessary to assure the community that the interviewers were there to describe the program in and of itself and not to select individuals who would support some perceived organizational agenda. Thus, the presentation of the purposes of the research does not finish simply with the introduction or pre-interview stage. Once the consultants begin participating in the interview, they may raise additional questions, and the research team will have to continually clarify the original purpose. It is also an opportunity to begin documenting contacts.

Interview Phase

After the contact phase comes the interview phase. Parts of this phase include the pre-interview phase, the interview proper, and the postinterview phase. The pre-interview phase involves introductions and an explanation of the purposes of that specific interview, and it concludes with whatever negotiations have to be made. In recent times, additional questions involve recorded-interview ownership and consultant privacy. Many organizations, such as the National Park Service, issue forms that each consultant needs to sign. These forms establish that the information to be collected is owned by the federal government and therefore is part of the public domain. The consultant is welcome to a copy of the recorded interview since it is part of the public domain. All other copies to other people will be redacted or in other ways screened for privacy. In short, the consultant needs to know up front that their rights to privacy are not necessarily the same as rights of confidentiality or anonymity. Finally, as outlined in Chapter 2, research conduct may be reviewed by IRBs or comparable organizations. It might be that whatever is agreed on with the IRB may have to be reconciled with the consultant. It is for these reasons that an interviewer needs to know what the relevant laws are before ever entering the field. Again, one should never promise what cannot be delivered. In the United States, the relevant laws are articulated in the Freedom of Information Act (1967).

Part of the negotiations may include the interview question itself. It is best to try to phrase the question in terms of what the interviewer *should* know rather than what the consultant *actually* knows. This question orientation is a way of easing into the consultant's expert knowledge without implicitly threatening to expose the consultant's imagined or possible ignorance. Asking what the interviewer should know is more indirect and less provocative, and it may even shift the responsibility of what to tell the interviewer onto the consultant. It stresses the consultant's control by asking, "Tell me what I should know and no more." It seems that even the most accomplished expert fears exposure and sometimes overcompensates by very aggressive talk. As experts, they know something the interviewer does not, so it is best to treat the consultant's knowledge with respect.

It also is best to expect the unexpected and be prepared to negotiate. The following interview between Oswald Werner and the noted anthropologist Victor Uchendu illustrates the need to be both systematic and flexible. Werner wanted to find out what kinds of "food" there are among the Igbo of Nigeria:

> **OW:** We are interested in the fact that in the Igbo version of the Lord's Prayer "our daily bread" back translates into English as "food." Can you tell us what the Igbo consider food?
>
> **VU:** Well, I suppose the usual things . . .
>
> **OW:** No, no, I don't want you to answer in English. Could you formulate a question something like, "What kind of things are food?" in Igbo?

VU: Sure, that would be, "Kedu ihendi Igbonaeri?" (What things the Igbo do eat?)

OW: Let me play back the question to you [plays recorder]. Would you try to answer your own question?

VU: [amused, after a long pause] You know that question cannot be answered, except in one way: Nri. That means, "everything that fills the belly."

OW: Interesting. Could we now formulate a question, again in Igbo, asking something like, "What kind of things fill the belly?"

VU: Sure, "Kedu ihe nwere ike iju afo?" (What things have can fill the belly?)

OW: I'll play it back again and would you like to answer it [plays back the question].

VU: [laughing] You know, it is funny, but that question cannot be answered except one way: Nri utra (pounded food). That means, "everything that is pounded." In West Africa, we pound our food in large wooden mom.

OW: Could we ask once more, "What are the things that are pounded?"

VU: Yes, indeed. "Dedu ih eji eme utaru?" (What things can make pounded food?)

OW: Now let me play it back again and you answer it. OK?

VU: [laughing hard] You know, that is the question you should have asked in the first place. The answer is, "Yam, manioc taro (cocoyam), and manioc products, especially gari."

OW: Don't the Igbo ever eat some stuff, like fruit or a banana, right off the tree without pounding it?

VU: Sure they do, but that is not nri or food—that is the phrase cham cham, or a snack. These are epe (orange), ahirika (banana), ube (tropical pear)—things that don't fill the belly—not even meat! They are in a class of foods that Americans call "snacks." Yam, plantain, taro, maize, and so on may be boiled, roasted, or fried. They are not classified as nri; they remain snacks. (Werner & Schoepfle, 1987a, pp. 320–321)

In a similar example, ethnographers interviewing Navajo students asked, "What kinds of students are there [in a reservation school]?" One student diffidently answered, "Oh, boys, girls, I guess; but they're all brown." The answer improved after the researcher explained the question more carefully, using illustrations of what students from other classes and schools had said. These other students distinguished among one another by attitudes toward classes or teachers, degree of language competence, clan, and other attributes. Referring to previous answers, of course, may have inadvertently biased the student, but at least it got her talking.

The Interview Proper

Within the interview proper, the researcher needs to keep track of three levels of control: formal, informal, and conversational. Information is gathered differently for each level. In the formal interview, the commencement of the interview is apparent. The researcher turns on the recorder and marks the formal beginning (we assume that a recorder is permitted). Before the recording, both the ethnographer and the consultant make themselves comfortable. Either one may get a pencil and notepad (or relevant electronic equipment) ready as they settle into the interview. During conversations following the formal interview, it is not unusual for the consultant to add information of importance to the researcher—even after the recorder is turned off. At this point, the ethnographer should ask the consultant if they may turn on the recorder to record the additional discourse.

In an informal interview, the beginning and ending are not always as clear as in a formal interview. Sometimes, an interview may happen simply as part of a personal encounter. During these instances, the ethnographer may ask the consultant if they can turn on their recording equipment, if it is nearby. There may be interruptions or movement between different sites. Some parts of the interview may be audio recorded electronically, while other parts are recorded in notes only. Similarly, other people may appear who happen to be in the vicinity of the interview and ask to be recorded. These kinds of informal interviews are much more likely to happen in the grass hut setting discussed in Chapter 2, but they have occurred in offices and other locations too.

Casual interviews result from casual encounters or conversations, and they have both advantages and disadvantages. They may often preclude a formal recording session. An ethnographer may walk around with a recorder turned on all the time. The advantages are that conversations are spontaneous and unaffected by the formality of an interview. However, they can be very intrusive since it is best to inform the consultant of an interview recording. Also, recall of unrecorded or incompletely recorded interviews can be problematic. Few, if any, ethnographers have the ability to recall verbatim. Issues such as those articulated by the *systematic distortion hypothesis* (see Chapter 1) also emerge here. To mitigate these problems, transcription may be necessary as soon as possible after the interview (Werner, 1999).

At the end of an interview, a researcher should be prepared to ask, "Is there anything that I should know that we have not talked about?" It is here that the consultant has a chance to add what—for whatever reason—nobody thought of asking.

Turn Taking in Interviews. As with any other verbal expression, answers to questions have a form and function. When any conversation—including an interview—proceeds, those involved have to take turns talking. "Turn taking" refers to the rules in any language that indicate when a speaker has finished talking and the listener is expected to begin speaking. Most languages and cultures have some kind of what can be called continuation attention markers (Werner & Schoepfle, 1993) or topic orientation markers (Fraser, 2009). When people normally listen to a lengthy explanation or long story, they indicate that they are still listening by nodding, smiling, or maybe saying something like "uh huh." These cues can be nonverbal or visual. One of the best ways to appreciate nonvisual cues is when two people are having a phone conversation and there is a long pause. Someone might ask, "Are you still there?" At that point, the other has to give a verbal cue indicating that they are still engaged in conversation.

For the interviewer, there is one other—often forgotten—marker: taking notes. One of my colleagues had observed me conducting interviews with Anglo consultants and pointed out that when I was taking notes, my note taking would lag behind the consultant's answers and not finish when the consultant had completed talking. There was thus a pause to which the consultant was unaccustomed. In response, the consultant would often fill up the silence with further information pertinent to the interview. I had not noticed this since I was too busy taking notes. Navajo consultants, on the other hand, when they had finished would simply wait quietly for me to finish writing.

Different cultures, in other words, have different practices for turn taking. For another example, when bilingual Navajo consultants were asked questions either in Navajo or in English, they would pause before answering. Inexperienced Anglo interviewers would become uneasy and begin rephrasing the question or in other ways filling up the silence. The Navajos, on the other hand, were doing one of two things: (1) they were either thinking through the question so that they could make a full answer, as if it were a verbal essay, or (2) they were forming an answer for themselves in Navajo and then thinking about how to translate it into English, their second language. In either event, the resulting disjunct would sometimes make both sides uncomfortable.

Also, to Navajos, it was important to speak in clearly articulated and complete bodies of verbal discourse, because it indicated that they had mastered the ability to think in an organized way (Begishe et al., 1981). It followed that the Navajo considered it highly unmannerly and disrespectful to interject questions during any pause. If they were talking with an Anglo, they would wait until the Anglo had completely finished speaking. An Anglo, on the other hand, is often more accustomed to a faster-paced, more frequent, give-and-take pattern in speaking. For Anglos, such a rapid give-and-take indicates interest on the part of the interviewer. To the Navajos themselves, this might indicate disrespect, a short attention span, lack of self-discipline, or in other ways an inability to listen to what is being said.

One final example of attempts to master Navajo turn taking by non-Navajos has its amusing pitfalls. Werner recounted how he had taken up the practice of responding to pauses in Navajo discourse—even if he could not follow all of it—by saying "mmm." This approach is used often by Navajos to show the speaker that they are following what is being said, and for the speaker to continue. Werner's interpreter, Kenneth Begishe, later observed to Werner that one of the consultants was stopping what he was saying in the middle of a sentence—clearly before he was finished. Werner, nevertheless, followed each pause by saying "mmm," much to the amusement of the consultant. Werner and Begishe both agreed that while the incident was amusing at Werner's expense, Werner was well within reason to err on the side of caution.

Postinterview

The postinterview phase involves both a business and a personal element. The business element consists of the ethnographer stowing away any equipment, thanking the consultants for their time and effort, and making payment if it was negotiated. The personal part of the postinterview often resembles a friendly visit rather than a business transaction. It may involve gossiping; discussing the news of the day; commenting on the progress of friends, children, and grandchildren; or other casual exchanges. As a general rule, the postinterview phase can become lengthier and be more likely to occur with repeated visits by the ethnographer.

This postinterview time may also be a time when friendships can develop. In this context, one is also advised to be very careful about accepting invitations for lunch or a meal after the interview. As a general rule, it is best to accept these offers. For whatever the reason, people might be offended if the interviewer does not accept. Normally, it is often best to watch what the translator or native coresearcher does and to follow along.

Much ethnographically important background information may also be exchanged during the informal post interview. In fact, this time may be seen as a casual interview. Statements tend to be spontaneous and more unguarded. These unguarded moments may afford time in which unexpected information comes to light, which is available to the ethnographer only in informal settings.

At still other times, the postinterview may be the time in which the interview continues but with the consultant turning the tables on the ethnographer. One of the consultant's questions may be a variant of "What is this research all about?" Even though the ethnographer may have explained the purpose to the consultant, it is obviously best to reiterate. Sometimes, a restatement clarifies things for the consultant, and in other circumstances, slightly different wording may bring up consultant insights previously not mentioned. Consultants may often not be sure of what the ethnographer is looking for and will ask further questions about the research. Another variant is "What have you found?" Or even "What have others told you?" Both may be answered by variants of "Here is what I have been told." It is then possible to provide whatever quotation or graphic representation may be appropriate. One may then bring the questioner back in with the rejoinder question "Did I understand all that right?"

In one example, I was interviewing some Navajo high school students about the kinds of students and activities there were in the school. This was part of the six ethnographies of Navajo schools (Werner et al., 1976) conducted by what was then the Navajo Tribal Division of Education. I was interviewing two sophomore high school girls at the same time because both maintained that they were too shy to be speaking with me alone. The interview did not proceed very well, and after about 20 minutes I decided to end the interview and, as usual, thank the students for their time and trouble. When I completed my polite attempt at an exit, one of the girls asked, "What are you trying to find out?" I decided to answer by describing the information I had obtained on the kinds of students described by others. While I was talking, I illustrated this description with tree diagrams on a sheet of paper. The girls responded by giving their own view of what this classification system looked like. An interview that almost ended in 20 minutes ended up lasting 2 hours. I then had to escort the girls back to their next classes and excuse their absence to their teachers. This example also highlights opportunities for verbal confirmation or disconfirmation of researcher conclusions or analysis. Almost any conversation between an ethnographer and a member of the culture being studied can be an interview.

Space

Grand-tour and mini-tour questions of space elicit the consultant's description of the stage on which they act and the boundaries of that stage. Descriptions include buildings, properties, features of landscapes, and the boundaries of all of these. Within these boundaries, consultants discuss how they define each scene, what they perform within it, and where they perform it. The grand-tour question about space becomes a walk or similar travel through the personal space of the consultant. The space can be as small as a room, such as in a Navajo school in *Six Navajo School Ethnographies* (Werner et al., 1976). It can be the landscape on which someone would lead an ethnographer and narrate all the things they do during a year or maybe throughout their lives (Fanale, 1982; Ritts-Benally, personal communication, 1984; Schoepfle et al., 1982). The answer to the grand tour may be a guided tour of an area. The consultant may recall the tour sometimes without actually being in the specific location, as in a white room or grass hut interview.

Once an interview about a landscape begins, memory involves associating concepts with physical locations. Thus, an ethnographer should capitalize on what appears to be a combination of sequence (e.g., Luria, 1969) and a simple use of land features as mnemonics (Harwood, 1976). As the interview progresses, the consultant may mention important information about other people, activities, feelings, judgments, and evaluations associated with the feature. The knowledge behind a consultant's narrative on a landscape is often inextricably interwoven with the other kinds of knowledge. As always, the ethnographer's best policy is to let the consultant talk. For example, Spradley (1974) recommended, especially when interviewing children, asking them to assume that the ethnographers are blindfolded and that everything must be explained in words. The same approach can be used effectively in actual walks through any kind of building.

In a narrated walk on a landscape, the consultant may neglect to mention visible features that may have been mentioned by other consultants or observed by the ethnographer. These omissions may offer important clues about the consultant's position in a social group, about their feelings and attitudes relating to these spaces or toward the occupants of these spaces during various times. Before jumping to any conclusions about the omission, the ethnographer should ask the consultant whether anything was missed. Or they may wish to take up the discussion with other consultants.

A useful tool that may help the consultant remember the features of a landscape and activities associated with it is a map. Hand-drawn maps are important since they may provide unexpected indicators of social organization, values, and other kinds of knowledge. They can also be strengthened by application of GPS (Jones, Drury, & McBeath, 2011).

Maps of Tlingit houses

I had an opportunity years ago to inspect some maps of Sitka, Alaska, drawn by Tlingit Indians in the 18th century. The houses were drawn smaller than the houses of the Russian colonists. Yet from other evidence, we know that the two house types were about the same size. A great opportunity was missed because no one saw the potential importance of questioning about the blanket and asking them why they felt that the colonists' houses were larger than their own. Such a follow-up question is clearly one that no longer qualifies as a grand tour, it's obviously a mini-tour. It focuses on the details of particular perceptions by the consultants. Without an interview, it is difficult to speculate today on what psychological meaning (if any) that the Tlingit attached to the relative size of the house drawings. (Werner & Schoepfle, 1987a, pp. 324–325)

Interviews about space can be one of the best opportunities for the ethnographer to act—very sincerely—as one ignorant of the consultant's knowledge. Spradley's (1974) recommendation to simulate the role of a blind person applies here as well.

The same approach can be used effectively in actual walks through any kind of building. I used a grand-tour approach to space while working at what was then the U.S. General Accounting Office (1994):

> My colleague Lawrence Solomon and I were led on a site visit tour of one of the surviving textile mills in North Carolina. We accompanied a group of state level U.S. Environmental Protection Agency pollution prevention program staff while they conducted a waste audit of the mill. The noise of the machinery was so deafening that everybody—the state pollution prevention staff, and even the employees at the mill—wore hearing protection. While the state staff appeared able to carry on a conversation with the employees, the GAO site visitors were unable to do so. Using a simple stenographer's pad, I simply sketched each of the places where state staff and employees stopped to talk. The notes included a crudely drawn map that described the physical properties of each location. The next morning, at what was supposed to be a short, perhaps 45-minute, exit interview, I proceeded to interview the staff. The interview elicited their recollections of what was discussed at each of the places where they stopped. Three hours later, the interview ended, and the staff shook their heads, and said, perhaps with more than a note of irony, "we didn't know we knew so much."

The answers, however, provided important information on the technical knowledge necessary for the staff to conduct the audit. I reviewed the conclusions with the staff, and they concurred.

A second kind of map includes those charted or digitized by government or commercial agencies. Included among these are today's digital and satellite maps. Other field manuals in anthropology deal directly with mapmaking, so only those aspects of mapping (Offen, 2003) that apply directly to cognitive ethnography are mentioned here. Distances, for example, can often be measured by walking and counting one's steps—something easily describable in human terms. It is important to consider how the natives might feel about such an activity carried out by the ethnographer.

Mapmaking can be threatening, especially to people who are afraid of excessive taxation or land use appropriation by outsiders. An ethnographer pacing up and down the fields of a village may thus provoke suspicion and hostility. It may even be dangerous to life and limb. On the other hand, ethnographers have encountered situations in which consultants see the ethnographer's careful pacing and measurement of land as indicative of their interest and of caring what the consultant has to say. Ultimately, the ethnographer must depend on common sense to keep out of trouble Herlihy and Knapp (2003).

Mapping serving the needs of peoples protecting their lands is well known (Herlihy, 2003a) Participatant mapping is a means of involving the consultants (Offen, 2003). According to Herlihy (2003), "participatory mapping in which local peoples are involved in the actual drawing of maps has become very widespread particularly in Latin America" (p. 303).

Maps of the interview itself may be sketched either by drawing or by graphing. For example, a drawing of an office may look like that shown in Figure 4.2.

Figure 4.2 Office Map

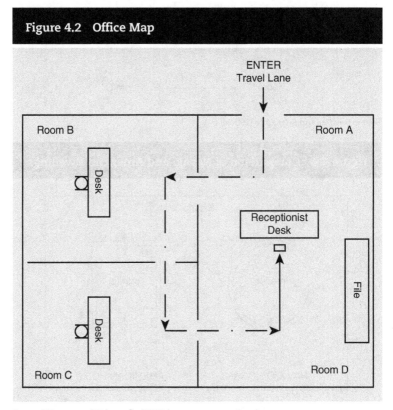

Source: Werner and Schoepfle (1987a).

The bold lines are walls, the open line segments are doors, and the traffic patterns are represented as dotted lines. Figure 4.3 shows the same office but graphing the office traffic.

The nodes represent interiors of rooms or sets. The lines represent traffic and possible directions of the traffic or communication.

Another variation of a mapping graph may look like a round hogan, the traditional Navajo dwelling, as shown in Figure 4.4. The figure compares it with a typical American home with a front and back entrance.

Figure 4.3   Office Map

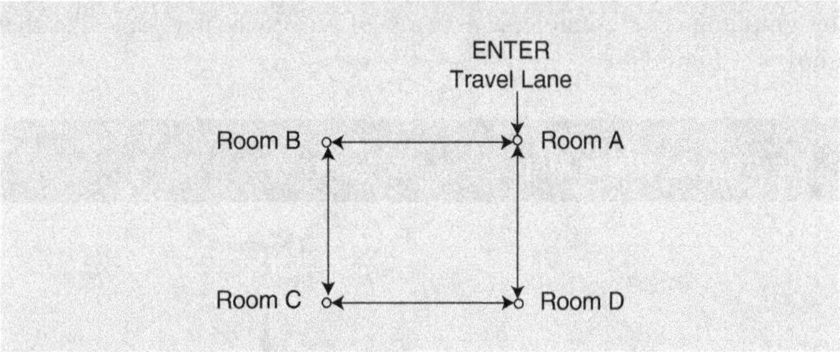

Source: Werner and Schoepfle (1987a).

Figure 4.4   Comparison of Navajo and American Dwellings

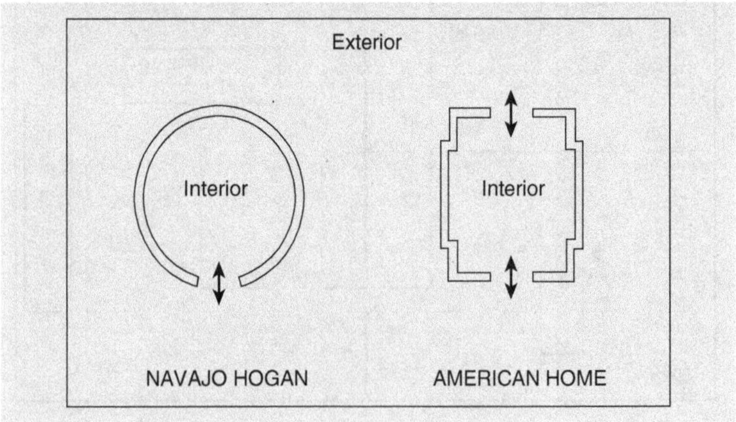

Source: Werner and Schoepfle (1987a).

In Figure 4.5, the traffic patterns translate as Venn diagrams. The exterior space is the universe, and the interior space one of the regions, or subset of a region. The interior/exterior regions can also be represented by graphs as in Figure 4.5. They are both graphic representations showing that there is only one possible way to get from inside a Navajo hogan to the outside, while there are two or more in the typical American home. The choice of which type of graph to use depends on what is being observed or described. Simple "topological" graphs can often lead to insights about behavior that can be missed in more complex maps. Thus, for example, the Hogan door is more strategically important than the front door of the American home.

The importance of land and space as a mnemonic is not difficult to understand. The ethnographer walks with the consultants and listens to them talk about locations and sites that are important in their lives (Fanale, 1982). Nabahe (Schoepfle et al., 1982) also used grand-tour questions of space to elicit and sketch the different ecological zones used by traditional Navajo livestock herders along the eastern side of

Figure 4.5   Comparison of Navajo and Anglo Houses, Stressing Entry and Exit

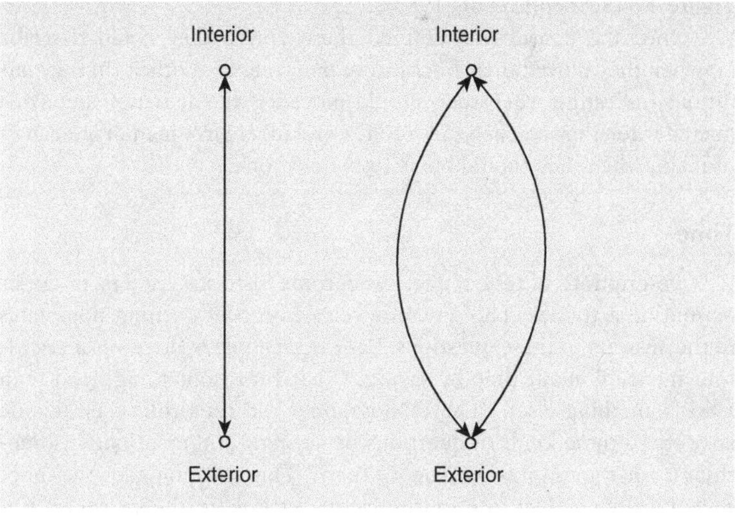

Source: Werner and Schoepfle (1987a).

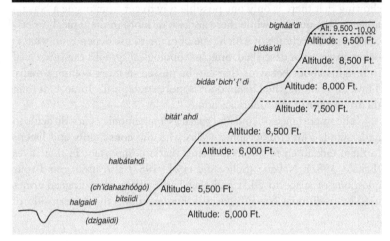

Figure 4.6 Ecological Zones Identified by Navajo in Seasonal Transhumance on the Eastern Side of the Chuska Mountains, New Mexico

bigháa'di Alt. 9,500 -10,00
Altitude: 9,500 Ft.

bidáa'di
Altitude: 8,500 Ft.

bidáa' bich'{' di
Altitude: 8,000 Ft.

bitát' ahdi
Altitude: 7,500 Ft.

Altitude: 6,500 Ft.

Altitude: 6,000 Ft.

halbátahdi

(ch'idahazhóógó) Altitude: 5,500 Ft.
halgaidi bitsíidi

(dzigaiidi) Altitude: 5,000 Ft.

Source: Nabahe.

the Chuska. The resulting descriptions could be illustrated as shown in Figure 4.6 (Schoepfle et al., 1982).

Once the consultants defined these zones, they could describe (a) when they moved their flocks from one zone to another, (b) the conditions indicating when they should move, (c) the activities they conducted when they reached these zones, and (d) environmental indicators of if and when they should move to the next one.

Time

Descriptions of time sequences become histories, careers, or cycles of routine activities. The semantic relationship of queuing dominates in the answers to these questions. Basically, people will answer a grand-tour question about time by saying, "First I do [something], and then I do [something else]." The ethnographer can then follow up on the answers to these kinds of questions by saying, "You mentioned [something]; what goes on when you do that?" This question adds the more semantically complex relationship of part–whole to the sequence. For example, turning off the alarm is part of waking up.

All people act in a temporal sequence. They act this way regardless of who they are and how they are involved in the social life being studied. The semantic relationship of sequence, or queuing, is thus exceedingly important. Sequence requires individuals to synchronize their actions with those of others around them. Grand-tour questions of sequence thus describe not only how to structure time but also to sequentially order tasks. In addition, they reveal the context in which individuals or groups are mobilized for certain tasks. Therefore, temporal sequences of activities may also provide the basis for individual social relationships. The fact that these sequences may occur on a regular basis becomes very important for understanding the cultural knowledge of peoples' social lives.

The most common temporal unit chosen for the first grand-tour question of time is the day, and it is perhaps the most popular. Nevertheless, there is nothing to prohibit the use of other units of time, such as the week, month, season of the year, or yearly cycle. There are, however, variations among the cultures encountered throughout the world. These include the boundaries of daily human activity and appear straightforward and universal.

A human activity day is not identical with the astronomical day—from sunrise to sunset—or the 24-hour day. Everyone requires sleep, so sleep offers the best boundary criterion. There is great variability in how long people sleep and whether or not their sleep is interrupted. Nevertheless, returning to an assigned sleeping place can serve as a reasonable, well-defined boundary of human activity. The day has additional methodological and theoretical importance and advantages. Methodologically, a day is of sufficiently brief duration to allow the ethnographer to compare observations with interview data. It is also possible to work out adequate sampling plans for interviews and observation. Readers interested in pursuing the day are welcome to read John Roberts's (1956) pioneering work on the Zuni daily activities and Martin Topper's (Topper, 1972; Topper et al., 1974) treatment of Navajo daily activities. Many articles have doubtless followed.

The yearly cycle may be just as important as the daily one, particularly for a society centered on agriculture or pastoralism. Thus, working out a yearly plan—particularly for nonurbanized societies—can be important for providing a framework within which comparisons are more easily drawn.

Finally, it is the regular recurrence of days, weeks, years, or other durations that makes the discussion of sequence for ethnography different from a discussion of history. History can best be seen as a sequence of unique events. Ethnographers are looking for patterns and routines. Thus, they expect the consultant to respond with all the possible activities they can perform at a given point in time and space, and how they may choose among them. The answer often veers off the strict temporal sequence of a particular activity and toward a description of all possible activities that may occur during a particular time. For example, consultants may describe smaller durations than a day. In short, these plans are outlines, not unique historical events. Similarly, the yearly cycle of activities may depend on the choices people make, depending on environmental and other conditions.

The difference between history and ethnography, however, does not mean that the elicitation of histories is antithetical to ethnography. In fact, some publications maintain that oral history is a kind of ethnography (National Park Service, 2004). Again, caution is required. First, historical or biographical descriptions tend to concentrate on the life of one person or what happened in one incident. These single units are not the core of ethnography. Nevertheless, there is an overlap. In an ethnographic interview, biographical and historical accounts are highly informative because they can be *case examples* or *case studies* of the recurring events and their patterns that constitute the ethnographic description. Similarly, if an ethnographer records a number of historical or biographical sketches, these too become the building blocks of ethnography. Nevertheless, history will require as distinct a factual anchor as possible in date, time, location, person, antecedent, and consequent. Ethnography requires these as well but must also recognize that legends, creation accounts, or tales are valuable if not so easy to anchor.

In one example, I was assigned to evaluate the petitions from a group seeking federal acknowledgment as an Indian tribe. Part of this evaluation involved determining whether there were recurring patterns of social interaction that might indicate the continued existence of a tribal community through time (25 CFR 83.7(b), 1994). From a review of other interviews, I had found that simply asking about the kinds of social relationships that existed or the interactions that might occur regularly often failed to yield effective answers. People reported feeling uncomfortable about giving answers that might be construed as not favorable to the evaluation of social interaction. As a result, the answers did not yield adequate details of who was interacting with whom. I therefore began every interview by asking petitioner members, "What are the important things that happened to you or that you did as part of your life?" Again, the person might often ask, "What do you mean by 'important'?" And I would answer, "Whatever is important to you." A single ensuing interview often lasted as long as an and a half. The answers yielded oral histories and personal biographies, which in turn yielded more information on the kinds of social interaction. The information included where, with whom, and when the activities occurred. From this information, I was better able to propose an evaluation of whether this interaction was indicative of an ongoing according to the regulations or simply indicative of commemorative activity.

People

People are placed third in this discussion because ethnographers may select a geographical location before knowing much about the people within the setting. This possibility is relevant whether the setting is a day care center, a school, a small village, or a livestock camp. At other times, the study may be a cross-sectional ethnography of warriors, the homeless, prostitutes, drug addicts, gang bangers, or students. In these instances, the first criterion of selection is one of several characteristics of the actors themselves.

Grand-tour questions about actors produce information similar to that provided by the cast list in a play, or perhaps a personnel file system. The actual grand-tour question may involve little more than a request for a list of people's names. It is then up to subsequent mini-tour questioning to elicit details about similarities or differences. Such detail may include titles, responsibilities, relationships, or other actors with whom the consultant must interact.

It may also include evaluations, feelings, and judgments about others. Likes and dislikes of others in one's surroundings are inevitable aspects of social life. Judicious ethnographers do not press their luck in field relations by delving too quickly into the likes and dislikes toward others. At first, it is safer to stick with the facts, such as roles or location in the identities of different people. Likes and dislikes can surface as a by-product of other interviewing, and often soon do so.

Answers to grand-tour questions about people often emerge spontaneously during the interview. For example, students in the Navajo schools in the *Six Navajo School Ethnographies* (Werner et al., 1976) freely mentioned the teachers with whom they had taken classes. It was only reasonable for the interviewer to then ask something to the effect of "You mentioned teachers; what kind of teachers are there in the school?" In some cases, the students would answer the question simply by listing the classes that they attended during the day. Sometimes, however, they would mention teachers they liked or did not like. From this, the interviewer could elicit information about what other kinds of teachers there were.

Interestingly, the students would sometimes answer the question by evaluating the effectiveness of the teacher in facilitating their learning. In other cases, they would emphasize how nice the teacher was to them or how easy it was to develop a rapport with the teacher. From these answers, the ethnographers hypothesized that the predominantly Navajo-speaking students in the Bureau of Indian Affairs schools valued teachers more according to the ease of developing rapport. In the state-operated public schools and the community-controlled contract schools, the students evaluated the teachers more on how well they taught the subjects. Subsequent survey research generated from these kinds of ethnographies (Blount et al., 2015) established significant patterns of likes and dislikes (Garrison & Schoepfle, 1977).

GRAND-TOUR AND MINI-TOUR QUESTIONS ABOUT PEOPLE THROUGH PERSONAL NETWORKS: THE CRYSTALIZED STRUCTURE OF A "SNOWBALL SAMPLE"

One kind of research question ethnographers at some point have to ask is "Who would be able or willing to talk to me in an interview?" Chapter 2 proposed this question when discussing plans for the early stages of making contact in a project. Here, we expand our perspective on networks from a sampling to a monitoring device. Werner (1989) explains ethnographic sampling by proposing a *sampling tree*. He derived this tree from a sample of people he interviewed as part of a study of gardeners in a Hungarian village. By diagramming the individuals interviewed, the kinds of interviews, and the contacts to other individuals interviewed, he could identify and keep track of all the people and the kinds of people he had interviewed. For example, he discovered that his sample included more men than women, although both were about equally involved in gardening. Thus, he was able to better balance his interview sample. Figure 4.7 is a tree diagram that shows how Werner identified individuals for interview. He could distinguish among groups of people whom he found were reticent about being interviewed (e.g., women), who had to be interviewed under special conditions, or who possessed special kinds of knowledge.

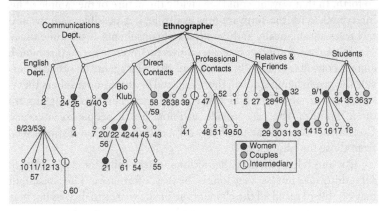

Figure 4.7 Tree Diagram of Werner's Network Sample

Source: Werner (1989).

This tree diagram gives ethnographers a working view of the representativeness of their sample, the kind of people reached, the extent of the network, and the paths of contact. The numbers 1 to 61 represent Werner's 61 interviews during 4 months of field work. Multiple numbers represent more than one interview.

The tree also shows that there are six avenues of access to consultants knowledgeable about gardens. Werner first contacted as consultants colleagues in the academic departments at Janus Pannonius University in southern Hungary. From there, he literally knocked on doors or met people casually through chance encounters. These opportunities came through his contacts with professional colleagues, relatives, and friends in Hungary and through students in his classes at the University of Pécs, Hungary. One of his more successful direct contacts occurred when he attended a meeting of the organic gardening club, the Bio-Klub. That gathering led to interviews with virtually every member. In each of these contact groups, there were key men and women who introduced him to still more people with gardens who were willing to be interviewed.

Although not marked in the diagram, Figure 4.7 reveals clues as to whether some of these individuals were rural or urban. It also shows how many young people, older people, couples, women, men, and so on, could be sampled. The diagram gave Werner a good overview of the representativeness, that is, the range, of his consultants' knowledge.

Werner used several copies of this tree as part of his research. He color coded men versus women, rural versus urban, younger versus older, and so forth. In that way, he could see vividly the nature of the sample of his interviews. With the software now available, it is possible to draw contact trees automatically and keep track of consultants at the same time.

In general, a contact tree also allows the interviewer to distinguish among consultants initially referred to them by agents or officials outside the group being studied, those selected by the ethnographers themselves, and those referred by other consultants. The outside agents are often the ones who can provide an initial list of people to interview. Consultants selected as the fieldwork continues can be distinguished from those initially selected.

An interview eliciting definitions, taxonomies, or sequences of something may not last very long or be very informative. The consultant may be able to recall all the elements he or she wishes to discuss but may not always be able to recall *important* elements. Similarly, the consultant may be located in environments, be involved with other activities, or be with other people the ethnographer may notice. Elements of space, time, and other people are thus important because (a) they will contain information that will have to be represented in the interview record and journal and (b) they are part of the grand-tour/mini-tour questions themselves.

CHAPTER 5

ETHNOGRAPHIC ANALYSIS WITH COMPLEX LOGICAL-SEMANTIC RELATIONSHIPS

I n outlining the MTQ schema, Chapters 3 and 4 showed how analysis of the semantic relationships in fact begins *during* the interview and shapes the interview itself. This chapter builds on Chapters 3 and 4 and demonstrates further analysis after transcription and translation have finished. Such analysis allows for the application of more complex semantic relationships. The term "complex" refers to any statement that depends on the truth value of another statement (Quine, 1941). Examples of such semantic relationships include *implication*, *requirement*, *causality*, and *part–whole*.

ENHANCING MTQ ANALYSES

Again, MTQ analyses include *modification*, *taxonomy*, and *queuing*. The illustration for the easily confused M and T is through defining a zebra as a horse (T) with stripes (M). Occasionally, the terms "attribute" and "attribution" will be used for modification, and the term "category" will occasionally be used for taxonomy. Also, the term "sequence" will be used for queuing. By displaying the basic semantic relationships, various enhancements can be made.

Composite Folk Definitions

Modification is the cement of the folk definition. As discussed in Chapter 4, a folk definition consists of a term modified by attributes. Attributes are words or phrases that tell the reader more about the term being defined. The process for constructing a folk definition is straightforward: (a) identify a term or phrase to be defined and (b) gather other words and phrases from the consultants that tell more about this term.

Chapter 4 also indicated how folk definitions proceed from interviews. It stressed that the easiest way is to elicit a folk definition from *a single consultant* during an interview, and it emphasized use of the slip sort and word association interviews. A second kind is called a *composite* folk definition. Here, the ethnographer develops the definition from the transcribed interviews with two or more consultants.

When an interview includes more than one person it is important to pay close attention to the accuracy of the elicitations at all times. The interviewer has to carefully compare and contrast attributes yielded by the individual speakers. The interviewer must pay attention to how individual speakers overlap and disagree. The following example is part of a study conducted in San Juan County, New Mexico (Tonigan, 1982). The study evaluated a proposal to combine two predominantly Navajo Indian school districts into one district distinct from the rest of the county. The two districts were Shiprock and Kirtland. The former is located on the Navajo reservation; the latter is located off the reservation. As part of this evaluation, a team of ethnographers interviewed Navajo students from both districts who would be combined into the proposed new district. While both districts were predominantly Navajo, the Navajos in Kirtland District were considered more acculturated than those in Shiprock District. The simple question was how the Navajos in either district viewed the situation. The answers show that the students had negative views of each other. We are indebted to ethnographic researcher Rose R. Morgan for these definitions.

The first definition is from the standpoint of the Kirtland students with regard to those in Shiprock. According to the Kirtland students, the predominantly Navajo-speaking Shiprock students appeared to go out of their way to make the Kirtland students feel ill at ease. Thus, the Kirtland students described the Shiprock students in this way.

Definition: Shiprock Students

1. They are hard to get along with.

2. They live in the old ways.

3. They eat traditional foods.

4. They speak Navajo, and many of us don't.

5. They are not nice to me.

6. They would say things in Navajo and give me funny looks.

7. I don't speak Navajo, and I don't see why they have to act that way.

8. They drink down there.

9. They get more homework there than they do here, but the students [there] fight a lot.

10. They even fight with teachers.

The second definition is from the viewpoint of the Shiprock students. It highlights the shared differences between the lifestyles of the two groups of Navajos.

Definition: Kirtland Students

1. I wouldn't be their friend if they were the last people on earth.

2. Anybody [who] goes to Kirtland is no friend of mine.

3. They call us Johns.

4. They feel that the kind of school and the kind of courses they have are better than the ones in Shiprock.

5. They say we are no good, that students here like to smoke and drink all the time.

Although the researchers identified only 5 attributes from the Shiprock students and 10 from the Kirtland students, the Shiprock definition is no simpler in construction. The public schools in *Six Navajo School Ethnographies* (Werner et al., 1976) showed that "Johns" were defined as students who (a) lived in the rural areas of the reservation, (b) lived in traditional hogans, (c) ate traditional foods such as mutton stew and fried bread, and (d) spoke predominantly Navajo. The latter attribute also indicated that these Navajos spoke English with a Navajo accent. As a result of these markers, they were often considered less intelligent and less knowledgeable about the urban life that was part of a normal public school student's daily life. The Shiprock students, in turn, indeed saw themselves as more "John" because they still had more ties with the Navajo reservation. Thus, the term when used by a Kirtland student carried a pejorative weight to it, but not so much so when used by Shiprock students among themselves.

Queuing and Verbal Action Plans

As explained in Chapter 4, any queuing phrase states that one action or perceived event occurs before or after another. It is diagrammed as follows:

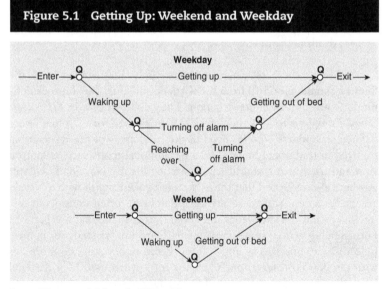

The directed line segments A, B, and C denote acts or events that occur one after another. The nodes, labeled as "Q," denote "and then." Verbs or verb phrases then label the names of the activities.

A VAP is an elaboration of queuing in two ways. First, it represents a recurrent sequence of activities in a body of cultural knowledge. It differs from a personal history because it is recurring. Nevertheless, both plans and histories can be diagrammed similarly in two principal ways (Werner & Schoepfle, 1987b). The first is through a simple list; the second is the graph, which is easier to follow. Figure 5.1 shows not only the weekday getting up shown in Chapter 4 but also a weekend variant.

Again, the arrows are labeled with the activities associated with getting up. They show a definite starting point (Enter) and a definite end point (Exit).

Figure 5.1   Getting Up: Weekend and Weekday

Source: Werner and Schoepfle 1987, vol 2.

As outlined in Chapter 4, the basic, or atomic, plan represents the barest semantic content of action verbs. This level of activity is known as an atomic plan because the consultant does not break down the detail any further. There are subatomic plans, but consultants are not always forthcoming in describing them because there is too much detail. Part of the problem of too much detail is that subplans are often in a *part–whole* relationship with the more inclusive plan. When the subplans and part–whole relationships are combined, the result is a VAP (see Chapter 4). It is the subplans that have fewer modifiers and hence are more atomic.

The reason for starting with the atomic plan, however, is that they are the least culture bound. This is true on the lowest level of a VAP. It represents a grouping or chunking of elements, often with universal notions. Comparing the Euro-American concepts of "weaving" with those of the Navajo shows how this similarly breaks down when examined in the greater detail involved in a VAP. For the activity of weaving, the *American Heritage Dictionary* (1969) reads, "to make [cloth] by interlacing the threads of the weft and the warp on a loom" (p. 1452). In the Navajo culture's weaving, the loom is upright and has no shuttle. The colored wool is threaded by hand between the vertical warp (Werner & Schoepfle, 1987b). The cultural implications of such a difference become dramatic when consultants describe the self-discipline that someone learning to weave must master. Navajo consultants have described how closely they had to pay attention to what they were weaving, which colors had to be used or combined, and the many times they had to practice or redo part of a weaving project until they had corrected it. Many of the women used to talk about how they quietly went out to a cornfield with their looms and practiced out of sight of others until they were satisfied with their performance. Both men and women Navajo coresearchers applied the same attitude in Navajo transcription learning. They would watch how their more experienced peers operated. No one would know if they were interested. Then, after a couple of weeks' absence, they would return to the research offices fully skilled in transcription. On returning, their research peers would joke about their having "gone to the cornfield."

Navajo planting activities further illustrate some cultural differences in VAP, from the standpoint of a more complex plan (Werner & Schoepfle, 1987b). The following example is of a complex plan, not an atomic plan.

For Traditional Navajos, planting starts in the center of the field, spiraling clockwise (sun wise) outward to the edge planting with a digging stick every three or 4 feet. Another important prerequisite of planting is the performance of appropriate planting prayers and songs. Planting may therefore be viewed as having two plans: a secular one for placing seeds in the ground, and a sacred one for performing the appropriate ceremonies that guarantee a good harvest. (Werner & Schoepfle, 1987b, p. 113)

ANALYSIS OF COMPLEX SEMANTIC RELATIONSHIPS

This book has skirted complex relationships. Examples of such relationships are part–whole, cause–effect, and requirement relationships. Other similar relationships can be found in Casagrande and Hale (1967).

Part-Whole

The part–whole relationship is difficult to define. For English speakers, the parts of the body are among the most common examples. The heart, for example, is a part of the body but is not a kind of body. In some languages, moreover, and for some children (Litowitz & Novy, 1984), this relationship is difficult to elicit. Also, the meanings translate somewhat differently in different languages. For example, the English phrase "the thumb is part of the hand" translates as the "hands have a thumb" in Hopi, in Navajo as the "thumb is at the hand," and in Rapa Nai "the thumb is a position of the hand" (Werner & Schoepfle, 1987b, pp. 84–85).

Moreover, eliciting elements of a part–whole relationship combines with other, atomic relations such as sequence. For example, in Navajo, the order of body parts recited in ceremonial contexts is strictly prescribed, beginning at the head and progressing to the feet. Similarly the part–whole relationship is indispensable in describing VAPs. The embeddedness of the part–whole relationship indeed becomes most dramatic when diagramming.

Another example is from diagramming thought in English. We have already demonstrated how to diagram part–whole as part of the sequence in VAPs. Part–whole can also be stated abstractly, in the form of "X is an aspect of Y." The concept of "thought" in English illustrates this (see Figure 5.2). For further discussion on this subject see D'Andrade (1983).

Another example, from the Rapa Nui, shows body parts (Figure 5.3).

Figure 5.2　Aspects or Parts of Western Thought

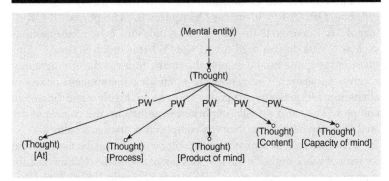

Source: Werner and Schoepfle 1987, vol 2.

Figure 5.3　Partial Tree of Rapa Nui Body Parts

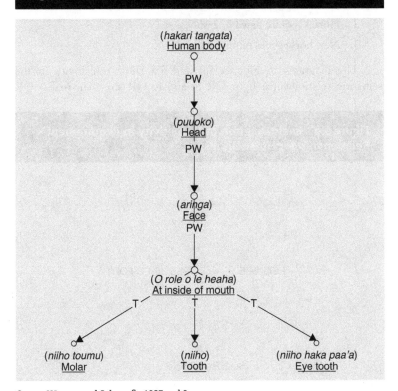

Source: Werner and Schoepfle 1987, vol 2.

Requirement Relationships

The requirement relationship can be represented by RQ and its reflexive, QR. "A RQ B" means "A requires B." The phrase "B QR A" means "B is required for A." This relationship generates questions such as "What do you need for A?" or "What is required for A?" This questioning frame can be reapplied as many times as the ethnographer receives an answer. The results are often long requirement chains of elicitation and generate structures that can be highly value laden and complex. They also provide important insights into the culture under study and can help schematize the complex processes in a culture.

As an example, we look at the adage "For want of a nail the shoe was lost, for want of a shoe the horse was lost, for want of a horse the rider was lost, for want of a rider the battle was lost" (Werner & Schoepfle, 1987b). This aphorism can be broken down into the following sentences, with RQ relationships:

1. Successful battle requires riders and horses.
2. Riders require horses.
3. Horses require new horse shoes.
4. New horse shoes require nails.

The diagrams in Figures 5.4 and 5.5 show transitivity in the semantic relationships: If (n QR c) and (c QR sb), then (nails) QR

Figure 5.4   Basic Diagram of Transitivity in Requirement Relationship for Horse Shoes

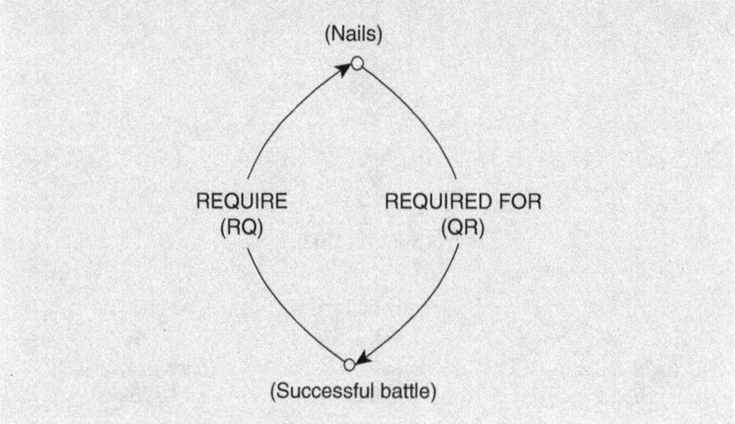

Source: Werner and Schoepfle 1987, vol 2.

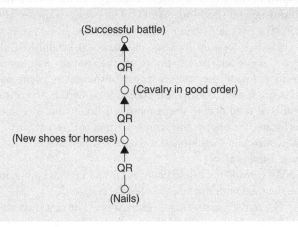

Figure 5.5 Alternate Diagram of Transitivity in Requirement Relationship for Horse Shoes

Source: Werner and Schoepfle 1987, vol 2.

(successful battle). The figures show that the relationships QR are transitive, and this transitivity enhances the ease of elicitation.

The inverse relationships of RQ and QR imply a *cause–effect relationship* as well. From our example above, Figure 5.4 shows that "successful battles because of nails," or "nails caused the successful battle." Figure 5.5 shows the equally true inverse statement. The major strength of the RQ/QR relation lies in its use as a point of intersection between other kinds of semantic relationships. It is equally capable of supplying insights into theoretical constructs, value structures, and the details of everyday living.

Causal Relationship

Little is known about how human beings talk about causation. Cause–effect is a complex relationship of the familiar canonical form "A is the cause of B,"

A ○──────is the cause of──────▶ B

or its inverse, "B because of A."

B ○──────because of──────▶ A

Causes, like taxonomy, part–whole, and plans, may form extensive lexical/semantic fields.

A study by Ahern (1979), cited in Werner and Schoepfle (1987b), serves as an illustration of how the analysis might work. Ahern investigated the reasons behind a strained relationship between the Navajos in the Tower Rock Community and the Lava Flow State Park Administration (fictitious names). The previous owner of the land on which the park had been recently established had allowed the Navajos to graze livestock on it. After the park was established, the area was fenced and declared off limits to the Navajo neighbors and their livestock. In addition, before its establishment as a state park, the land was a site for the concession booths used by the Navajos to sell fried bread and food during the annual Fall Rodeo and Ceremonial, which was located nearby. At the same time that the park was established, the Fall Rodeo and Ceremonial were moved permanently to another site about 5 miles away.

We provide the causal diagrams of the various complaints as a tree-type diagram with the lines labeled as "because."

The tree diagrams are self-explanatory. The first diagram (Figure 5.6) shows the overall results of the research. The succeeding tree diagrams then elaborate on certain details within the first, overarching one.

Figure 5.7 represents a part of a larger tree that explains in detail each of the five elements in Figure 5.6. It elaborates on how the pow-wow has changed unfavorably for many of the local Navajos.

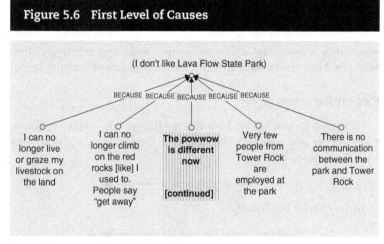

Figure 5.6   First Level of Causes

(I don't like Lava Flow State Park)

BECAUSE BECAUSE BECAUSE BECAUSE BECAUSE

| I can no longer live or graze my livestock on the land | I can no longer climb on the red rocks [like] I used to. People say "get away" | The powwow is different now [continued] | Very few people from Tower Rock are employed at the park | There is no communication between the park and Tower Rock |

Source: Werner and Schoepfle 1987, vol 2.

Figure 5.7 Second Level of Causes (re Powwow Is Different Now)

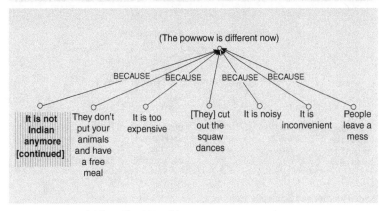

Source: Werner and Schoepfle 1987, vol 2.

Figure 5.8 Third Level of Causes ("It Is Not Indian Anymore")

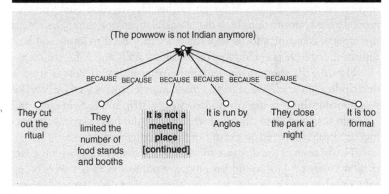

Source: Werner and Schoepfle 1987, vol 2.

Figure 5.8 provides additional information about the second-level element, "It is not Indian anymore." It gives more detail about why the Navajos think that "it is not Indian anymore."

The park management no longer permits them to engage in traditional activities such as sharing mutton or using the area as a site for

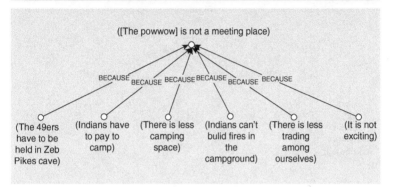

Figure 5.9 Fourth Level of Causes ("It Is Not a Meeting Place")

([The powwow] is not a meeting place)

BECAUSE BECAUSE BECAUSE BECAUSE BECAUSE BECAUSE

(The 49ers have to be held in Zeb Pikes cave)

(Indians have to pay to camp)

(There is less camping space)

(Indians can't build fires in the campground)

(There is less trading among ourselves)

(It is not exciting)

Source: Werner and Schoepfle 1987, vol 2.

squaw dances. At the same time, with a more diverse group of people using the area, it is more difficult to clean up after visitors from outside the Tower Rock area. Figure 5.9 shows the effects.

In all, these trees provide a well-organized visual structure for the impacts of the state park. Although further investigation could provide more detailed information about the causal relationships, the analysis helps the report's consumers focus on what more they need to know and how future ethnographers could focus on obtaining additional information.

Figure 5.10 shows a final example of causality. It comes from a description of the effects of forced resettlement experienced by Navajos neighboring those being confronted with a strip mine. Schoepfle and his team sketched out a model of what he and the Navajo coresearchers had been told occurred as a result of the resettlement.

The bottom of the diagram shows that the model starts with the fact that "we were told we would have to leave our home." They were being told, in other words, to relocate. The Navajos first described the immediate effects of being told to move: giving up sheep permits and their land, and living among strangers with whom they had few or no close relations. Higher levels show that they lost their sheep permits, they had to live among strangers who had no knowledge of their past leadership and public life, they had no public standing, and their children tended not to visit them. They then describe how the loss of sheep and land made it impossible to raise their children through example. They became lonely, depressed, and overwhelmed by a sense of shame for

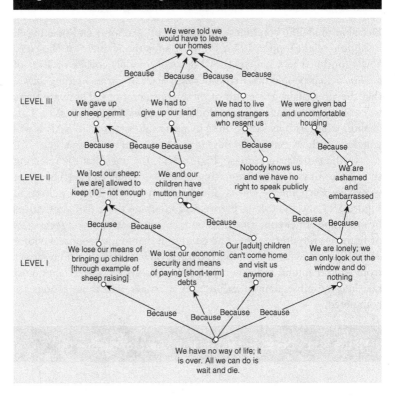

Figure 5.10 Causal Diagram for Forced Resettlement

ever having gone along with the demand to move. The model helps make sense of the conclusion—"All we can do is wait and die"—and the severe depression often accompanying relocation (Scudder, 1973, 1979; Topper, 1980).

This causal model is highly simplified and raises as many questions as it answers, and it is thus ethnographically useful. It shows immediately that there was no single set of trade-offs or mitigations to coal company development and its attendant resettlement. From the Navajo viewpoint, certain conditions would have to be met before others could be considered. If these inputs were placed into a decision model framework, such a process for mitigation—from the local Navajo viewpoint—could be considered. Application of decision models will be discussed in the following section.

ETHNOGRAPHIC DECISION MODELS: ENTERING CHOICE INTO VAPS

Decision modeling combines the analysis of taxonomy and queuing in a single model (Topper, 1976, 1980). It adds the element of choice to VAPs (outlined in Chapter 4). All decision models consist of a set of *conditions* that people must consider and a set of corresponding *actions* that they must take as a result of these considerations. There are three ways of diagramming decision models: *trees, flowcharts,* and *tables*. This chapter will start illustrating these by using the "getting up" VAP. It will conclude with an example of buying spices for Indian cuisine.

In the getting up exercise, Figure 5.11, the consultant is referring to a choice of two routines: getting up on weekends and getting up on weekdays. Each alternative was illustrated separately. The flowcharts in Figure 5.11 and the tree in Figure 5.12 combine these two alternatives by including either condition diamonds and alternative action rectangles or branches for alternatives. The condition diamonds propose a choice a person must make and answer the question with a yes/no. The arrows from each diamond indicate the specific actions the consultants must take and the subsequent questions they must ask once those actions are completed.

Figure 5.11   Decision Model Flow Chart for Getting Up

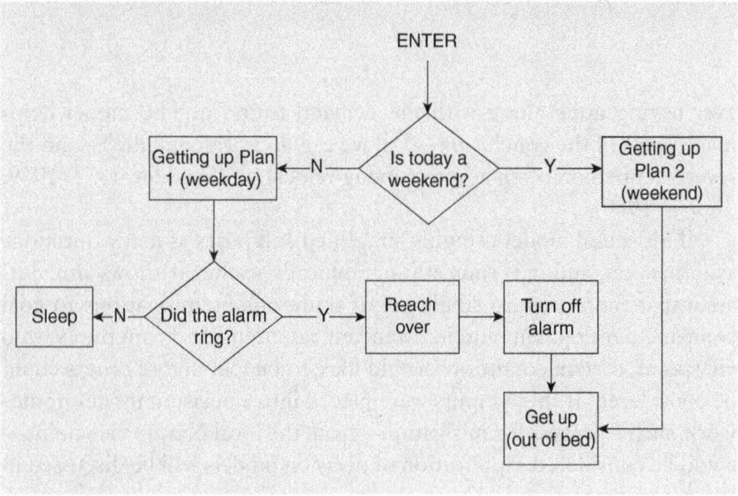

Source: Werner and Schoepfle 1987, vol 2.

The decision model flow chart combines into a single model the information of the two earlier diagrams of weekday/weekend (Figure 5.1). These two options can be collapsed into a single model. Figure 5.12 represents this flowchart for getting up as a *decision tree*. Here, the consultants again answer questions denoting conditions. Just as with the flowchart, the lines Y or N split and point to specific dichotomous choices.

Following these activities, the *arrows* point to the next addressable condition or activity. The nodes denote decision choice points.

Figure 5.13 represents the third kind of decision-making diagram, the *decision table*. It consists of four major elements: condition stub, condition entry, action stub, and action entry.

Figure 5.12   Decision Tree for Getting Up

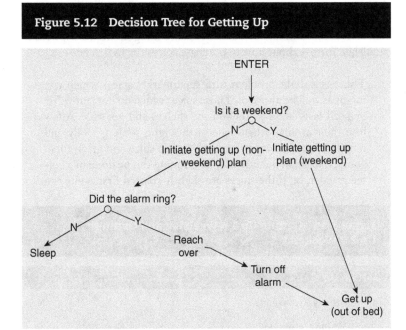

Figure 5.13   Basic Parts of a Decision Table

Condition Stub	Action Stub
Condition Entry	Action Entry

Source: Werner and Schoepfle 1987, vol 2.

The *condition stub* refers to the conditions the consultant has to consider before deciding to take action. The stub is phrased as *questions* such as "Is dinner ready?" or "Has Mother returned from the store?" They are answered with a yes/no. The *condition entry* contains the *rules* by which each condition is evaluated. If the condition is applicable, "Y" for "yes" applies. Otherwise, "N" for "no" applies. The *action stub* contains a list of the possible outcomes or actions. The *action entry* contains an "X" if the answer is "yes" or is blank if the answer is "no" (Figure 5.14).

While it is more detailed and involved, the decision table furnishes an excellent tool for ensuring that the entire universe of decision rules and outcomes has been developed and can be tested. The following example, purchasing spices, illustrates this. Again, the three kinds of diagramming are compared. This example was originally discussed in Werner and Schoepfle (1987b). It is an excerpt from a book by Madhur Jaffrey (1975)—and is a reasonably ideal ethnographic description, in published form—about how to purchase spices for Indian cuisine.

> There is a slight problem with supermarket spices which you might as well be aware of. Those spices which do not "move"— i.e., sell fast—tend to stay on the shelves and get stale. A few lose their aroma, others fade in the light, some get oily and rancid. Therefore try to buy only whole spice and grind them yourself in small quantities. The grinding can be done in a coffee grinder, or, if the spices are slightly roasted first, some can

Figure 5.14 Getting Up 1 = Weekday and Getting Up 2 = Weekend

Getting Up		1	2	3	4
1	Is today a weekend?	Y	Y	N	N
2	Did the alarm ring?	Y	N	Y	N
1	Getting Up Plan #2 (Weekend)	X			
2	Sleep		X		
3	Getting Up Plan #1			X	
4	(when awake) Weekend Plan				X

Source: Werner and Schoepfle 1987, vol 2.

be crushed between waxed paper with a rolling pin. The electric blender will grind spices, if you do them in sufficiently large quantities. If all else fails, you could use mortar and pestle, though that tends to crush spices rather than grind them. Whole spices retain their flavor for very long periods. Make sure you store them in jars with tightly screwed lids, well away from dampness and sunlight. Ground cumin and coriander are fine if bought from Indian spice dealers in small quantities. (Jaffrey, 1975, in Werner & Schoepfle, 1987b, p. 130)

The first step to diagramming this paragraph as a decision table is to number each sentence:

Slight problem with supermarket spices

1. There is a slight problem with supermarket spices which you might as well be aware of.

2. Those spices which do not "move"—i.e., sell fast—tend to stay on the shelves.

   a. A few lose their aroma.

   b. Others fade in the light.

   c. Some get oily and rancid.

3. Therefore try to buy only whole spice and grind them yourself in small quantities.

4. The grinding can be done in a coffee grinder.

5. Or, if the spices are slightly roasted first, some can be crushed between waxed paper with a rolling pin.

6. The electric blender will grind spices, if you do them in sufficiently large quantities.

7. If all else fails, you could use mortar and pestle, though that tends to crush spices rather than grind them.

8. Whole spices retain their flavor for very long periods.

9. Make sure you store them in jars with tightly screwed lids, well away from dampness and sunlight.

10. Ground cumin and coriander are fine if bought from Indian spice dealers in small quantities.

Figure 5.15   Tabulation of All Conditions and Actions

	Condition	Actions
1	Are the spices stale?	Buy and grind spices yourself.
2	Do you have a coffee grinder?	Grind in coffee grinder.
3	Do you have a rolling pin?	Roast slightly, grind with rolling pin between waxed paper.
4	Do you have a blender?	Grind in electric blender.
5	Do you have a sufficiently large quantity of spices?	Buy spices in the supermarket.
6	Do you have a mortar and pestle?	Use mortar and pestle.
7	Is the spice whole?	Buy spices whole.
8	Do you need cumin and coriander?	Buy from Indian spice dealer in small quantities.

Source: Werner and Schoepfle 1987, vol 2.

After tabulating the sentences, the next step is to examine each sentence and determine whether it is a condition or an action. They can be summarized as shown in Figure 5.15.

The next step in the analysis is to show how the sentences can be parsed into corresponding pairs of conditions and actions. It is often helpful to start with a flowchart (Figure 5.16) or decision tree (Figure 5.17) before proceeding to the tables.

Both the flow chart in Figure 5.16 and the decision tree in Figure 5.17 demonstrate that these models *combine both taxonomy and queuing* (Topper 1976, 1980). This combination allows ethnographers to factor the element of choice into the analysis of any behavior. The models are relatively easy to follow, and they allow the ethnographer to make quick sense of what the consultants describe. Although they may both appear very different from the decision table, either form generally translates smoothly into a decision table. However, reviewing these diagrams will highlight the uncertainties in understanding what Jaffrey

Figure 5.16   Decision Model Flow Chart for Buying Spices

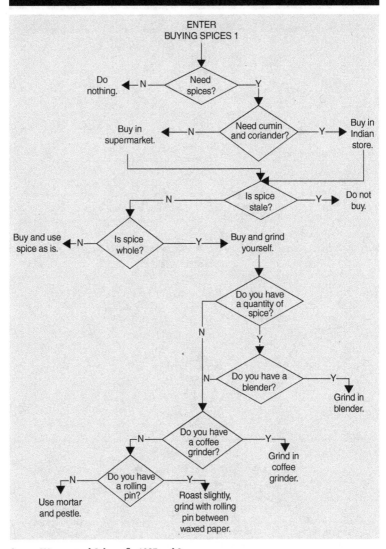

Source: Werner and Schoepfle 1987, vol 2.

really means. While applying these problems may sometimes be frustrating, they make possible the rigor necessary for an unbiased understanding of a cultural knowledge system. They help ensure that conditions and outcomes have been considered, and they ask more questions.

Figure 5.17 Decision Tree for Buying Spices

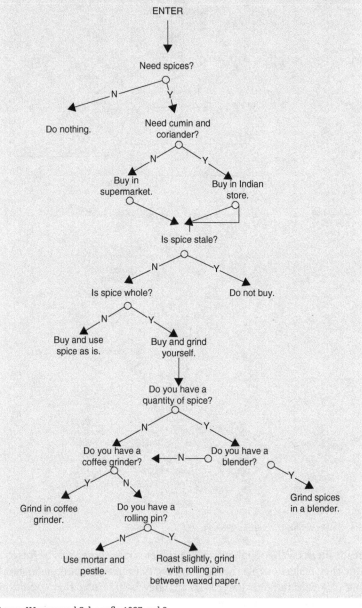

Source: Werner and Schoepfle 1987, vol 2.

Figure 5.18 Overview: Decision Table for Buying Spices

Buying Spices		1	2	3	4	5	6	7	8	9	10	11	12	13	14	15	16
1	Need spices?	Y	Y	Y	Y	Y	Y	Y	Y	N	N	N	N	N	N	N	N
2	Need cumin–coriander?	Y	Y	Y	Y	N	N	N	N	Y	Y	Y	Y	N	N	N	N
3	Are spices stale?	Y	Y	N	N	Y	Y	N	N	Y	Y	N	N	Y	Y	Y	N
4	Are spices whole?	Y	N	Y	N	Y	N	Y	N	Y	N	Y	N	Y	N	Y	N
1	Buy and grind yourself			X													
2	Buy in Indian store				X												
3	Do not buy	X	X														

Source: Werner and Schoepfle 1987, vol 2.

To generate decision tables, the first step is to interchange the rows and columns of the initial tabulation in Figure 5.15. Several questions immediately arise. First, the eight conditions and actions total 2^8, or 256, possible combinations. It would be best to reduce the possible combinations for the decision table to fit on an 8.5- by 11-inch piece of paper. The reason for this reduction is to make analysis simpler in the field.

Another problem is that knowledge about some conditions is incomplete. Since the ethnographer in this scenario cannot consult directly with the consultants, it will be necessary to make explicit some assumptions in every analysis. An examination of the data suggests that it is possible in this case to split all the original condition and action tables into two parts. Conditions 1, 7, and 8 in Figure 5.15 deal with the initial conditions of whether or not one needs to buy spices and whether to buy spices at a supermarket or buy cumin and coriander at the Indian spice store. The remaining conditions (2–6) deal with the question of what to do once the spices are purchased and brought home. This demonstration will concentrate on the first part, how to buy spices.

The chef can purchase cumin and coriander at the Indian store if they are needed. In addition, the ethnographer could assume that any other needed spices can also be bought at the Indian store. If the spice is whole, it must be ground at home. Again, to be safe, an ethnographer would normally check this with the consultants. There is also an implied sequence between the first two conditions, where to buy spices (supermarket or Indian store), and the last two conditions, which are concerned with whether they should be purchased or what to do with them once they have been purchased.

The ethnographer may decide in turn to split Buying Spices into two smaller tables: Buying Spices Part 1 (Figure 15.19) and Buying Spices Part 2 (Figure 15.20). In the Part 1 table, if the chef needs cumin

Figure 5.19 Buying Spices Part 1

Buying Spices: Part 1		1	2	3	4
1	Need spices?	Y	Y	N	N
2	Need cumin and coriander?	Y	N	Y	N
1	Buy in Indian store	X		X	
2	Buy in supermarket		X		
3	Do nothing				X

Source: Werner and Schoepfle 1987, vol 2.

and coriander, a trip to the Indian store is inevitable. However, if only spices other than cumin and coriander are needed, then they can be bought at the local supermarket.

In Buying Spices Part 2, another assumption is necessary. If the spice is neither stale nor whole, then it is all right to buy, although the spice will need to be ground at home since it is whole.

While the original Buying Spices decision table was simplified by breaking it into smaller parts, additional simplification may be possible by examining the tables for redundancy. A decision table contains a redundancy if two possible sets of conditions (columns) with the same outcomes have a different outcome for any one condition. For example, in Buying Spices Part 2, if the spice is stale, then it does not matter whether or not it is whole or ground, because the chef does not purchase the spice. The process of looking for redundancy in a decision table is called the *reduction process*. This process is represented schematically in Figure 5.21.

Figure 5.20 Buying Spices Part 2

Buying Spices: Part 2	1	2	3	4
1 Is spice stale?	Y	Y	N	N
2 Is spice whole?	Y	N	Y	N
1 Do not buy	X	X		
2 Buy and grind yourself			X	
3 Use as is				X

Source: Werner and Schoepfle 1987, vol 2.

Figure 5.21 Reduction Rule

Reduction Rule	1	2		1/2
1 Condition Number 1	Y	Y		Y
2 Condition Number 2	Y	Y		Y
3 Condition Number 3	N	Y	reduces to	—
4 Condition Number 4	N	N		N
1 Action Number 1	X	X		X

Applying the reduction rule to Buying Spices Parts 1 and 2 yields the tables in Figures 5.22 and 5.23.

The final reduced combination, in sequential order, is shown in Figure 5.23.

The same procedures can now be applied to the second half of the decision model, which is left to the reader as an exercise.

Figure 5.22   Application of Reduction Rule

Reduction Buying Spices Part 1	1	3		1/3
1 Need spices?	Y	N		—
2 Need cumin and coriander?	Y	Y	reduces to	Y
1 Buy in Indian store	X	X		X
Reduction Buying Spices Part 2	**1**	**2**		**1/2**
1 Is spice stale?	Y	Y		Y
2 Is spice whole?	Y	N	reduces to	—
1 Do not buy	X	X		X

Source: Werner and Schoepfle 1987, vol 2.

Figure 5.23   Final Reduced Sequential Buying Spices

Buying Spices Part I	1/3	2	4
1 Need spices?	—	Y	N
2 Need cumin and coriander?	Y	N	N
1 Buy in Indian store	X		
2 Buy in supermarket		X	
3 Do nothing			X
Buying Spices Part 2	**1/2**	**3**	**4**
1 Are spices stale?	Y	N	N
2 Are spices whole?	—	Y	N
1 Do not buy	X		
2 Buy and grind yourself		X	
3 Use as is			X

APPLYING DECISION MODELS IN COGNITIVE ETHNOGRAPHY

Ethnographic decision models have been applied in two principal ways. The first is to develop models that can validly predict observable behavior. The second is to test the validity of the stated preferences. The first is illustrated through a study by Ryan and Bernard (2006) on beverage can recycling. The second is based on the Navajo study of environmental impact mitigation preferences (Schoepfle, Burton, & Begishe, 1984; Schoepfle, Burton, & Morgan, 1984). First, both relied on cognitive ethnographic interviewing to understand what the people knew and believed. Second, they also developed and tested the models based on decision criteria derived from ethnography. Third, they validated and then tested the models on a wider sample of the population.

The beverage can recycling study involved using cognitive interview to gather information on the kinds of conditions that would encourage or discourage recycling. The resulting model in Figure 5.24 shows how the taxonomy and queuing sequenced the criteria.

Figure 5.24   Abbreviated Model Decision Tree for Recycling

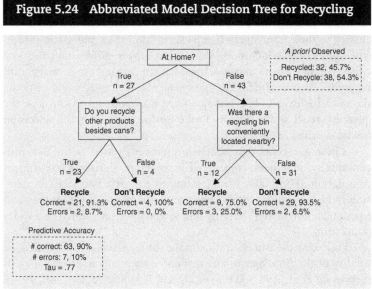

Source: Ryan and Bernard (2006). Reproduced by permission of the Society of Applied Anthropology from Melissa Cope

The figure also represents the results of the third stage, testing the tree on a new sample from a population with whom they had already conducted interviews. Finally, they tested their decision tree on a totally new sample of individuals. Those results are also shown in the figure.

In the second example, the Navajo team developed a model that articulated preferences toward certain outcomes. It tests preferences by simulating the order in which certain preferences were stated, albeit under political uncertainty. It was based on the kind of insight obtained from the causality model of what people knew about loss of land (see Figure 5.18).

This model, in effect, showed the order in which preferences had to be demanded before mitigation could be feasibly achieved (Figure 5.25). They were eliciting, in other words, a realistic model of what Navajos would like to do, under their present politically uncertain circumstances. No one knew whether or not the conditions would exist for supporting the mitigations. This decision model appears as follows. It is activated by answering yes/no to the question "Will the company make demands?" (*Da'lheejin hadajigédígiish t'áá aaníí kéhah nihídajókeed?*). The coal interests were "making demands" (i.e., proposing to mine coal and requiring the affected Navajos to relocate). The Navajo response was "We too can make demands" (*Nihi hanii doo'ádadii'níída*), which activated the decision model. If the answer to their interrogative requests is "no," then negotiating stops, with the Navajo conclusion "We can no longer think about this as a collective" (*doo bee adaanitsídeekeesǫda*). No demand can be made until its predecessor is satisfied. If the answer is "no" to any one of them, the model is exited. The Navajos were not prepared to consider the question at all and thus would take no further action. The decision model is exited in any event.

These questions represented preferences stated as the demands community members considered reasonable during a contingent negotiation. The Navajo team followed the first two steps in decision model design by interviewing and adjusting. However, they had to establish the model's validity and see how well it applied to a wider population.

Following the administration of the survey, the team established the validity of the flowchart model through entailment structural analysis (Schoepfle et al., 1981; White et al., 1977; White & McCann, 1981). Because of the variability of attitude and experience in the Navajo Nation, they also isolated and tested for factors such as education, traditional

Figure 5.25 Descriptive Decision Model Flowchart of Navajo Preferences

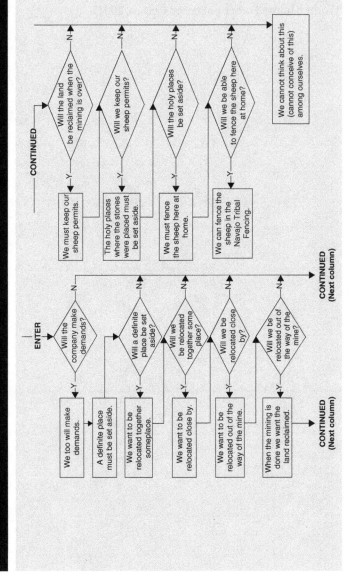

ENTER

Will the company make demands?
— Y → We too will make demands.
— N →

A definite place must be set aside.

Will a definite place be set aside?
— Y → We want to be relocated together someplace.
— N →

Will we be relocated together some place?
— Y → We want to be relocated close by.
— N →

Will we be relocated close by?
— Y → We want to be relocated out of the way of the mine.
— N →

Will we be relocated out of the way of the mine?
— Y → When the mining is done we want the land reclaimed.
— N →

CONTINUED (Next column)

CONTINUED

Will the land be reclaimed when the mining is over?
— Y → We must keep our sheep permits.
— N →

Will we keep our sheep permits?
— Y → The holy places where the stones were placed must be set aside.
— N →

Will the holy places be set aside?
— Y → We must fence the sheep here at home.
— N →

Will we be able to fence the sheep here at home?
— Y → We can fence the sheep in the Navajo Tribal Fencing.
— N →

We cannot think about this (cannot conceive of this) among ourselves.

CONTINUED (Next column)

grazing rights, and location. The research team applied canonical correlation analysis to establish the validity of the categories and then tested them. The distribution of the attitudes denoted by the model could then be tested through canonical correlation analysis (Schoepfle, Burton, & Begishe, 1984, or further information on how these mitigations affected World Bank and other policy see Cernea, 2002).

CHAPTER 6

LANGUAGE TRANSCRIPTION AND TRANSLATION

P revious chapters have stressed the need for cognitive ethnography to rely on the language of the consultant, and the consultant's knowledge. This reliance on the native language highlights the need for careful audio recording and transcription. Audio recording is where the ethnographer starts and the ethnography ends. So far, the illustrations of methods and results have stressed English or English translations. Much of the ethnography—even cognitive ethnography—can be in the language of the ethnographer. Nevertheless, the discussion on transcription, and especially translation, will direct attention to situations in which the language of the ethnographer is different from that used comfortably by the consultant. This section will highlight some of the pitfalls in making sure that interview recordings and their transcriptions will be clearly understood.

INTERVIEW TRANSCRIPTION

All interviews need to be transcribed. Thus, a *phonemic* transcription system should be in place. A language's *phonemes* are *all* and *only* those sounds that a language's speakers make and recognize as significant to conveying meaning. *Phonetics*, on the other hand, directs study toward *all* the sounds possible in human languages. Each language relies on only a few of these sounds to be understood. All other sounds are either babble or not considered distinguishable by the language speakers.

Phonetic Versus Phonemic

Phonetic orthographies are widely available but are far too cumbersome and unreliable to in most ethnoraphies. The principal reason is that these sound lists fail to factor out *allophonic* variation. That is, native speakers in any language may have slightly different ways of pronouncing certain sounds in different phonetic environments, but this does not confuse the native speaker. An outsider trying to write out a language phonetically would have no ability to distinguish which sound differences are meaningful to a native speaker and which are not.

Another reason is that transcribers using a phonetic system will be using different symbols for different sounds that the native speaker would consider to be the same. Examples abound. In English, the "t" sound varies by its location in a word. Its sound in the middle of a word, for example, "bottle," differs from its sound at the beginning of a word, such as "top." For English speakers, both sounds are represented by the letter "t" as the same phoneme.

An ethnographer thus needs to have an orthography, or a phonemic alphabet, in place. The orthography should include characters that represent *all and only* those sounds that convey meaning to speakers of the native language. These sounds, in turn, should be combined in a way that allows the writing of words and phrases recognizable by a variety of native speakers.

Today many languages have more or less "official" orthographies. The term "official" can stand for orthographies that either are recognized by a broad range of people in a society or have been adopted by the society's government, educational system, communities of respected intellectuals, or religious organizations. The ethnographer should use the system of writing with which most of their consultants are familiar. Some of the best sources about written languages are publications from missionary organizations. Linguist Kenneth Pike and the Summer Institute of Linguistics have trained many missionary linguists who are skilled in reducing an unwritten language to its phonemes. While missionary systems are not always highly regarded in certain societies, it may nevertheless be necessary to rely on their orthographies if no other exists.

The creation of a phonemic transcription requires special training. However, if none exists, a well-trained linguist should be able to construct a reliable inventory of phonemes. The average number of phonemes is about 30, but it could range from as low as 13 letters for Hawaiian to more than 60 for Abkhazian (see Hewitt, 1987). It is always valuable to consult with a linguist when analyzing an unwritten language. A word of caution is in order. The orthography proposed by the linguist should be designed to be easy for the transcribing keyboarder.

Recorded Interview Transcription

Many ethnographic interviews in the United States rely on a single language and orthography. Rapid transcription of these interviews introduces new problems. For example, a recorded interview may contain many pauses, incomplete sentences, unfinished thoughts, or interjections such as "uh" or "um." Some anthropologists and linguists have maintained that such incompleteness can be an indication of cognitive or psychological states that may have to be taken into account when analyzing the interview. For example, an incomplete or interrupted statement may be an indication of uncertainty in knowledge or some confusion in expression. From a sociolinguistic standpoint, these interferences may point to important information about the speaker, their knowledge, or their understanding of the interview question.

On the other hand, such thoroughness has its problems. First, it is not clear whether half starts, stammers, or other such interference will have any, other than speculative, value in understanding the context of what a speaker means. Insufficient time and attention may be available during fieldwork. Second, and perhaps more important, some consultants will be given transcripts of their interviews to review. They may not want to see or hear themselves speaking with imperfect phrasing or diction, and would like to sound articulate.

The ethnographer is thus in an uneasy position. On the one hand, they would like to be accurate; on the other, they would like to be considerate of the speaker. Striking a midpoint is not always easy, but it is possible. While circumstances may differ, one approach is to transcribe an interview with as many free-flowing sentences as possible while making a concerted effort to preserve idiosyncrasies in diction, expression, or understanding. Maintaining this balance involves consideration of both the researcher's individual style and the consultant's oratorical style.

Journal Transcription

Another aspect of transcription is how to transcribe the ethnographer's journal quickly and thoroughly in order to preserve the observations. We recommend a two-stage approach. In the first stage, the ethnographer dictates handwritten field notes or unwritten recollections into a digital recorder. In the second stage, the ethnographer listens to what was recorded and keyboards or types it into the journal. In each stage, the ethnographer can add observations or recollections into both the oral recording and the written entry. These notes may still not reflect a complete recollection of the day's events or interview (see Chapter 7), but they are helpful in that direction.

Transcription into English or a related language can be greatly helped through the use of speech recognition and transcription software, such as Dragon Naturally Speaking®. Here the ethnographer can listen either to themselves or to the consultant. Then, they can read what they have heard orally into the computer. Where usable, the transcription rate can be doubled, especially if the software has been well installed or "trained" to transcribe what the user dictates.

In either case, the ethnographer/transcriber needs to make a transcription of the recorded interviews. Since most digital recorders/playback machines mark the timed position of the interview, the markings need to be entered into the transcription, preferably within the text. Such entries should be made ideally every 5 minutes. Transcriptions should rely on the tracking in the digital recorder. Nothing can be worse than trying to find a phrase or statement for verification by having to listen through an hour's worth of interview.

Finally, the ethnographer needs to keep the consultant in mind after the interview. Some consultants highly value having copies of their interviews, for any number of personal, professional, or legal reasons. Interviewers under these circumstances have often provided digital recordings to people through CD/ROM, thumb drives, or similar memory devices. Many legal systems have mandated that the consultant be provided with the only complete, unredacted copy of an interview. All other copies need to be provided within the limits of the relevant statute. As implied in Chapter 2, the ethnographer should be prepared either to assume or to find out the legally and interpersonally appropriate actions.

INTERVIEW TRANSLATION

In many kinds of social science research, translation is too often taken for granted. Insufficient funding or attention is devoted to the quality assurance in this process. The ideal alternative to translation is for the ethnographer to develop fluency in the Native language. Achieving this goal, however, takes time and great effort, and both can be in short supply. Furthermore, "fluency" does not mean that the ethnographer is equally fluent in all cultural domains (see Chapter 1). Translation thus serves as both a bridge to understanding by the ethnographer and a part of research documentation.

Translation conveys meaning from the *source* language transferred into the *target* language of the ethnographer, usually in written form. Thus, any meaning in one language should be translatable into a close equivalence in another language—at least in theory—given sufficient space and time.

Two Kinds of Bilingualism

There are two kinds of bilingual language speakers: *coordinate bilinguals* and *compound bilinguals*. The former can speak, in our example, either Navajo or English. However, they cannot translate Navajo into English, and vice versa. The latter are capable of translating because they can understand and compose phrases in both languages that have similar or equivalent meaning. The process of translation can be represented as the comparison and recall of two versions of a word, a sentence, or a text in the languages of a *compound bilingual speaker*.

A bilingual individual relies on his or her memory to draw on memorized knowledge to make meaningful phrases in either language. They go through a process that allows them to remember and think in two languages. It is this process that is of interest. This kind of translation involves morpheme-by-morpheme analysis. Morphemes are minimally understandable grammatical parts of a language. The different kinds of translation are exceedingly important. We start with a step-by-step translation. Should the student wish for further detail, consult Werner and Schoepfle (1987a).

Step-by-Step Translation

The basic question is "Can the ethnographer or translator make a translation they can trust?" Or more precisely, "Can they make a translation that can be back-translated to the original?" Keeping track is difficult because many languages have a different word order from the English word order. When translating ethnographic texts not used for grammatical analysis, it is thus helpful to number every word in the source language and number the corresponding words in the final smooth target version. This numbering helps a reader unfamiliar with the source language to get some insights into the structure of the source language. The Navajo texts in this book follow this numbering convention.

Navajo: (1) *Asdzání léi'* (2) *yiltsą́ągo* (3) *bináál* (4) *łééchąą'í* (5) *halgaigi* (6) *ahééhádááh* (7).

Direct translation: A (2) woman (1) when she was pregnant (3), in her presence (4) a dog (5) in a field (meadow, open area) (6) was walking in a circle (7).

Free translation: In the presence of a pregnant woman, a dog was walking in circles in a field.

Then, all unnecessary translations of source morphemes are eliminated. The following example represents the more serious problem of how to represent a Navajo disease in Navajo knowledge, rather than simply translations of Western disease categories into Navajo. As Werner (1993) explains further, "Martha Austin-Garrison, working as co-principal investigator with Oswald Werner on the Navajo Ethno Medical Encyclopedia (NEME) project came across such a list of almost 100 items. One of the terms in the list was *Awéé' łééchąą'í yeełt'é*" (Werner & Schoepfle, 1987a, p. 365).

While the translation was complete enough for the purpose of the encyclopedia, Werner and Austin-Garrison began an ethnographic analysis for further understanding (Werner, 1993; Austin'Garrison, 2017 (11-13)). They began with a folk definition of the phrase *Awéé' łééchąą'í yiltsą́ągo yeełt'é*. Again, Austin-Garrison's translation into English begins with lengthening the Navajo. This length is not surprising given the nature of the differences between the two systems of cultural knowledge. The corresponding numbered translation and folk definition on which Austin-Garrison traced this translation follows. Note that the Navajo term *yiltsą́ągo* (pregnant) is removed initially.

Definition: *Awéé ' łééchąą'í yeełt'é*

Navajo: Asdzání (1) *léi'* (2) *bináál* (3) *łééchąą'í* (4) *halgaigi* (5) *ahééhádááh* (6).

Direct translation: A (2) woman (1) in her presence (3) a dog (4) in a field (meadow, open area) (5) was walking in a circle (6).

Navajo: Átséédą́ą́' (1) *shį́į́* (2) *łééchąą'í* (3) *ayói* (4) *ahoníłtéelgo* (5) *ahééhádááh* (6).

Direct translation: At first (1) it seems (2) the dog (3) was walking in a circle (6) in a very (4) wide area (5).

Navajo: Wónáásdóó (1) *áhoołts'íísígo* (2) *ahééhádááh* (3), *áko* (4) *názhnél'įįh* (5) , *jiní* (6).

Direct translation: Later (1) it was walking around (2) in a circle (3) in a small area, thus (4) she looked at it (now and then) (5), they say (6).

Navajo: Wónáásdóó (1) *tsxı̨́ı̨́łgo* (2) *náábał* (3).

Direct translation: Finally (1) it was going around (rotating) (3) fast (2).

Navajo: Hááhgóóshı̨́ı̨́ (1) *náábałgo* (2) *bitsee'* (3) *yótsa'go* (4) *naa'anátłish* (5).

Direct translation: Somehow (1) as it was gyrating (2) as it was holding in its mouth (4) its tail (3) it repeatedly was falling over (5).

Navajo: T'áá (1) *ákǫ́ǫ́* (2) *sitı̨́ı̨go* (3) *haashı̨́ı̨́* (4) *nízah* (5) *nináházhish* (6).

Direct translation: Just (1) there (2) it was lying (3) who knows (4) for how long (5) (a time) (6).

Navajo: Áádóó (1) *nínáádii'nah* (2) *dóó* (3) *nitsaago* (4) *ahééhádáahgo* (5) *yaa nínáádiidááh* (6).

Direct translation: And then (1) it [would] get up (2) and (3) [while] in a wide (big) (4) circle it [would] be walking (5) it [would] begin doing it again (6).

Navajo: Díí (1) *łééchąą'í* (2) *haashı̨́ı̨́* (3) *nízah* (4) *nihoolzhiizhgo* (5) *daaztsą́* (6).

Direct translation: This (1) dog (2) [while] for who knows (3) for how long (4) a time [it did it] (5) died (6).

Navajo: Asdzání (1) *ashchı̨́h* (2) *dóó* (3) *biyáázh* (4) *ts'ídá* (5) *naakits'áadah* (6) *binááhaigo* (7) *índa,* (8) *t'ah* (9) *nít'éę́'* (10) *biyáázh* (11) *níléí* (12) *halgaigi* (13) *ayóó* (14) *ahonı̨́łtsohgo* (15) *ahééhádááh* (16).

Direct translation: The woman (1) gave birth (2) and (3) [when] her son (4) was about (5) twelve (6) years old (7), then (8) suddenly (8, 9) her son (11) there (12) in a very (14) wide open area (13, 15) was walking [around] in a circle (16).

Navajo: Wónáásdóó (1) *t'áá* (2) *áhoołts'íísígo* (3) *ahééhádááh* (4).

Direct translation: And then (1) he walked in a circle (4) [in] just (2) a smaller [and smaller] area (3).

Navajo: T'áá (1) *názhnél'įįhgo* (2) *wónáásdóó* (3) *tsxįįłgo* (4) *náábałgo* (5) *naa'iigo'* (6) *dóó bikee'* (7) *yótą'* (9).

Direct translation: Just (1) as she kept looking (observing) him (2), finally (3) [while] quickly (4) gyrating (5) [and while] he fell over (6) and (7) he held (9) his feet (8).

Navajo: Haashįį (1) *nízah* (2) *nihoolzhiizh* (3) *sitįįgo* (4) *dóó* (5) *nídii'na'* (6).

Direct translation: Who knows (1) how long (2) (a time) (3) [after] he was lying there (4) and (5) he got up (6).

Navajo: Haashįį (1) *nízah* (2) *nihoolzhiizh* (3) *sitįįgo* (4) *dóó* (5) *nídii'na'* (6). *Dah náádiidzá* (1) *hótsaago* (2) *ahééhádáahgo* (3) *yaa nínáádiidzá* (4).

Direct translation: He began walking again (1) in a wide area (2) [and] walking in a circle (3) he did it again (4).

Navajo: Bimá (1) *dóó* (2) *bizhé'é* (3) *áni* (4), *haalá* (5) *yit'éego* (6) *nihi'awéé'* (7) *ákót'į?* (8) *ní* (9).

Direct translation: His mother (1) and (2) his father (3) spoke thus (4) "How come (5) our baby (7) is acting (6) in that way (8)," they said (9).

Navajo: Áádóóshįį (1) *biyáázh* (2) *nidadilniihii* (3) *yich'į'* (4) *bił* (5) *naaskai* (6).

Direct translation: And then it seems (1) with (5) her son (2) they went (6) to (4) a hand-trembler (diagnostician) (3).

Navajo: Ashkii (1) *bá* (2) *na'idéékid* (3) *nít'ęę'* (4) *łééchąą'í* (5) *ná'ooljiłí* (6) *yeełt'é* (7), *jiní* (8).

Direct translation: The boy (1) was (4) diagnosed (2, 3) that he "resembled" [his spirit was bothered by] (7) a dog (5) that had rabies (kept turning around) (6), they say (8).

Navajo: Łééchąą'í (1) *ná'ooljiłí* (2) *bá* (3) *ánályaago* (4) *doo át'įį da* (5) *silįį'* (6), *jiní* (7).

Direct translation: The dog (1) that had rabies (2) that ceremony they performed (4) for him (3) [and] he became (6) [such] that he did not act [that way again] (5), they say (7).

This added narrative gives the reader still more of an idea of the meaning of the definition derived from the translation. In addition to the narrative given above, Austin-Garrison discusses further:

> When you say, "*Awéé' łééchąą'í yeełt'é*," a Navajo will understand this easily—you have in your mind a picture of what is wrong with the baby. But when you say it to a modern doctor, he has no idea. To him, this is a culture sickness.
>
> The word *yeełt'é* is the key word, and it's very tough to translate it. It's easy to translate it literally, but the understanding of it, the meaning of it, is pretty hard. Literally, it means that you almost have to tell a whole story to get the whole thing across. I can't find one single word right now to fit that particular word. I'll tell you a story so you can try to get in your mind what it is I am trying to say. This whole statement refers to when the baby is still a fetus—in the womb.
>
> The pregnant woman or the expectant father, if he does something, like to the dog, in this case, *łééchąą'í*, to a dog if he kills a dog or if he in some way makes a dog suffer and the dog dies from the suffering—for instance, like one statement that usually comes up is when the father to the baby, *awéé',* that is going to be born, if he goes and hangs a little puppy by the neck with a wire, hangs it from a tree, and then hits it and tortures it and then it takes a long time for the puppy to die, and then he burns the whole puppy, that's real torture, you know, if you harm the animal.
>
> Somehow the spirit of that puppy harms the fetus in the mother's womb. Because the fetus in Navajo is considered very weak and doesn't have any supernatural or spiritual power, has no breathing of its own, lives totally by the mother's, you know, the child's life, spiritually. So the child is infected spiritually from the puppy.
>
> So say, the baby is born then, maybe the baby is growing up, from birth to however old—twenty years or, thirty years old . . . maybe he's hurting all over, and so he goes to the doctor and he says, "I have a neck pain." The neck may be all right. He may have a pretty good neck and . . . [a] modern doctor will say, "Oh, there's nothing wrong with you. It's all in your mind. I don't see anything wrong with you." And he'll keep going

around and say, "I have a very painful neck. The doctor says there's nothing wrong with me."

Finally he decides to go see a medicine man or a diagnostician, and the diagnostician will say, "Oh, you were still in your mother's womb. Your father tortured a little puppy and killed it and that's causing you to get pain in your neck. The way he tortured it was he hung the little puppy and beat it or shot it or however, tortured it with rocks, so you have aches and pain all over your body, because the wire that was around the puppy, in a way is around your neck now and you're suffering." (Werner, 1993, p. 12)

That's what "*awéé' łééchąą'í yeełt'é*" means.

We also hope we have shown, at the least, that an accurate translation enhances ethnography and confers greater understanding. However, translation is difficult and cannot be taken for granted. We now turn our attention to more abbreviated kinds of translation.

When Time (and Usually Money) Is of the Essence

Any researcher must be able to track the process well enough to be reasonably sure that the translated words or phrases in one language can be traced systematically back to the original. This is the justification for numbering. For a long speech, however, the numbering of words we have demonstrated here will be overwhelming. The following example shows how the wherewithal for this tracking can be maintained. It shows an efficient use of interpretation and how revisions of the interpretation can at least be negotiated, if not determined.

The speeches were recorded from local Navajo political representatives and education leaders who testified to the needs voiced by their constituents and parents in their communities. Hearings were held and reported in schools and chapter houses throughout the Navajo Nation, close to the homes of the people who were testifying. The testimony needed to be translated into English and published for review throughout the United States, including what were then the Department of Health, Education, and Welfare and the Bureau of Indian Affairs, as well as the U.S. Congress.

The publication process proceeded with the following steps. First, the testimony was recorded in Navajo, the primary language of the political discourse. Next, a small studio was set up with two recording devices: The first one played the already recorded Navajo hearings testimony; the second one recorded both the playback of the hearings testimony and the English translation of the testimony, phrase by phrase. Third, the Navajo Division of Education staff transcribed the testimony in its English version.

While this process appeared "low-tech," it had significant political results. First, it showed a diversity of easily accessible Navajo parent views on the education of their children. This testimony also could be shared by other Navajo and non-Navajo education officials among the three different school administrative systems (see Chapter 1).

The translation and English-language transcription processes gave validity to the hearings and established them as representing the attitudes of the parents and their aspirations for their children beyond those reported by various education agency surveys. The hearings also represented the carefully considered Navajo political process throughout the reservation. For example, some who gave testimony occasionally disputed what the translated version showed. They were invited to the offices to review the original Navajo tapes and the translation of their testimony. Then, they were given the opportunity to work with the Division of Education staff to clarify and correct any testimony where necessary.

The hearings thus formed an important basis for subsequent educational policy planning. The translation process helped a segment of Navajos and non-Navajos to understand the viewpoint of people, many of whom had made a considerable effort to confer with fellow community members and think through what they were going to say. In research generally, the ethnographer will not always have the time and equipment for direct, step-by-step translation.

CHAPTER 7

OBSERVATION

A mong the different kinds of observation, participant observation has emerged as the most common approach in ethnography (DeWalt et al., 1998). The fact remains that *the first activity any ethnographer will undertake on arrival at a new site is to observe*. This chapter highlights some of the limitations of systematic observation and how it can be related to cognitive ethnography, particularly by having knowledgeable consultants involved.

PROPOSED JUSTIFICATIONS FOR SOLE RELIANCE ON OBSERVATION

Anthropologists John and Beatrice Whiting (1970) proposed a number of situations in which observation would be the only means of obtaining information. Werner and Schoepfle (1987a) have considered many of these reasons as artifacts of how fieldwork has been conducted in the past, and not always a reflection of the inherent limitations of the consultant's knowledge. The following subheadings summarize the justifications for sole reliance on observation.

No Term Exists in a Specific Language

The first reason often given is that no term exists in the native language for a given idea. For certain microbehaviors, such as sawing wood, drilling, walking, or maintaining adequate boundaries in personal interaction (Hall, 1969), eliciting specific terms may be indeed difficult. Such knowledge may be tacit (see Chapter 1) and may be too cumbersome for members of a social group to teach verbally, either through translation or through technical vocabulary.

However, there are often ways of getting people to discuss some kinds of nonverbal interaction indirectly. One example is from proxemics, or the maintenance of personal space. Here, people may not be able to describe a specific spatial orientation, but they can describe when they are uncomfortable with somebody getting too close to them or otherwise acting inappropriately (Hall, 1969). Similarly, there may not be a specific word, but there may be phrases that can enlighten the ethnographer. The very least an ethnographer should do is ensure that *assuming the absence of any vocabulary in a language is done only after a very careful examination of the resources in that language* (Werner & Schoepfle, 1987a).

The more different a language is from the ethnographer's syntax or meaning, the more dangerous the assumption of absence becomes. One of the best examples of this difficulty comes from Werner and Schoepfle (1987a) on the absence of the term "color" in Navajo:

> Much has been made of the absence of a general term for "color"; some investigators use it as evidence for a lack of abstraction in Navajo. We discovered quite by accident that while color is not indicated in Navajo taxonomies, speakers of the language have available to them a considerably more abstract and general term. The Navajo word in question *ánoolinígíí*, can best be translated as "surface appearance" or "surface phenomena of an object." In addition to color, this concept includes texture (spotted, striped, variegated, etc.), and other qualities of surfaces. Thus the statement that the Navajo have no cover term for color is misleading. Using this as evidence for a lack of abstract thought, is false and even vicious. (p. 267)

Observation can be very appealing because it spares the ethnographer from making contact with strangers. As a result, deficiencies of vocabulary are often reported simply because no one has bothered to ask about them. A good example comes from the Navajo anatomical terminology:

> In a survey of Indian health service physicians' perceptions of Navajo anatomical knowledge, Leighton and Kennedy (1959) reported that the Navajo have an "impoverished" anatomical terminology. In the *Anatomical Atlas of the Navajo* (Werner et al., 1986), we found over 500 anatomical terms. Previously, nobody had taken the time to systematically query

knowledgeable Navajos about their knowledge of anatomy. (Werner & Schoepfle, 1987a, p. 267)

Also, an ethnographer should never take too seriously the often quoted distinction between explicit and implicit (or hidden) categories in any language. It is often possible to find people in any culture who can make generally implicit ideas explicit. The average native may not know—or only vaguely perceive—why certain ceremonial activities must be performed in a certain way. A knowledgeable expert may exist somewhere among the cultural group.

Certain Kinds of Behavior Do Not Exist

A second major excuse for not interviewing is the assumption that no clear or generalized pattern of behavior exists in the cultural group. However, consultants themselves may simply not talk about a behavior not because the behavior does not exist but because they may not have been exposed to it. If there are subgroups within a culture or internal variation within the group, some consultants may not always know. It is thus important to select consultants who are highly knowledgeable and have a reputation as such. Finally, if there is no generalized pattern of behavior, one must ask how people predict one another's actions. How do they interact across subgroup boundaries at all? In effect, the assumption that there is no behavior pattern is itself a potentially fascinating subject of research. This does not justify assuming that none exists.

Certain Behavior Cannot Be Verbalized

A third justification is the assumed inability of the consultant to verbalize certain behavior. If consultants cannot verbalize their behavior or the behavior of others in a particular domain, the first reaction by the researcher should be to suspect that the consultant was inappropriately chosen. Somebody has to know. In most other cases, the discrepancy may be due to the ethnographer's ignorance of values. In a strange culture, it is always safer to assume the ignorance of the ethnographer than that of the consultants.

As an illustration, anthropologist Emile Scheppers (personal communication, Werner & Schoepfle, 1987a, p. 269) described how he was unable to elicit anatomical terms in his classifications from Hopi consultants. Then he explained to them that his ignorance was comparable to that of a child's attempt to learn. He was able to convince his consultants that they should treat him as if he were a Hopi child. Soon thereafter, he was able to elicit the desired information without difficulty.

Sensitive Subjects: Beating Around the Bush

A fourth reason given involves reporting on behavior that may be inappropriate. This difficulty suggests that in some cultural domains direct questions are often unanswerable. It does not mean lack of knowledge. Kenneth Begishe explained to an inexperienced Navajo interviewer how to obtain information on Navajo beliefs about death. Since this is an area that is fraught with supernatural danger, a traditional Navajo will be very circumspect in talking about these matters. Begishe thought that it was best "to beat around the bush" with indirect questions. "If you keep beating around the bush," he said, "eventually you'll discover what it is in the bush" (personal communication, Werner & Schoepfle, 1987a, p. 270).

Embarrassing Situations

A similar justification is that the subject matter or the interview circumstances are too sensitive for the consultant to discuss. Ethnographers have always experienced interview situations in which they sense that the consultant feels uncomfortable about talking. However, there is little or no evidence showing that observation yields any better information than interview in these situations. The safest policy is to take the time and effort to build relationships of mutual trust and privacy and to subject all observations to confidential comment by trusted consultants. At the same time, there are situations in which the better policy is to abandon a sensitive topic or delay asking questions about it until a better understanding and trust are established. The intent here is not to negate the need for observation. Rather, it indicates the need to reconcile observation with consultant interviews, instead of abandoning interviews altogether.

KINDS OF OBSERVATION

This section addresses observation itself in greater detail. Many books have considered many different kinds of observation. The authors have found three kinds of observation most helpful: (1) Spradley's method, (2) the journal recording of the ethnographer, and (3) recorded observations, such as photography.

Spradley's Process of Systematic Observation

According to Spradley (1980), a systematic approach requires that the observer understands the social group under study. He proposes three levels toward achieving systematic observation: descriptive, focused, and selective. Descriptive observation appears quite early in a study and is the least systematic. It has a form of shotgun approach, in which the observer records everything he or she sees and hears. It is valuable, however, because the poorly understood minutiae of one observer may be an important topic of discussion for someone else. Or its importance may emerge later in the research, after the ethnographers review their notes.

The focused observation is more systematic because the ethnographer and the consultants have had an opportunity to comment mutually on the observation and the explanation of certain behavior. Focused observation, according to Spradley, is parallel to the structural, often taxonomic questions that are used as a follow-up to what has been observed. In Spradley's (1980) study of waitresses, for example, he observed waitresses receiving tips and could ask a taxonomic question such as "What are the different strategies for getting tips?" The basic point is that through such questions the researcher is forced to include the consultant's comments and descriptions in the focused observation.

Selective observation is the most systematic. Unlike the others, it focuses on the attributes of different activities, not the whole activity itself. In the above citation of Spradley (1980), the question is not focused on the strategies themselves for obtaining tips but, rather, "What are the different *kinds of* strategies for obtaining tips, and how do they differ?" Spradley's schedule of the three observation types is very important precisely because it shadows the ethnographic interview approach (see Chapter 4).

Micro-ethnographic observation, a variant of this approach, is favored by those advocating some kinds of "mixed-methods" research. Here, small units of behavior are often codified, and their frequency distribution can be aggregated into various kinds of socially significant units. This book acknowledges the efficacy of these approaches, but *only* after a consultant has explained his or her understanding of these units. Generally, "emic" students of behavior, such as linguist Kenneth Pike (1967), have advocated description of these patterns. However, the units of behavior can be understood only by their place within these patterns.

The Journal

The journal is a repository of an ethnographer's observations and experiences, uninformed by the consultant. It also includes impressions of the ethnographer's surroundings. In some cases, the journal includes the ethnographer's feelings or internal psychological or emotional states. The general literature contains many examples of intimate internal observations, including the journals of Malinowski (1967), and the letters of Franz Boaz (Rohner, 1969). There are also the retrospective memoirs of Ruth Benedict (Mead, 1966), Hortense Powdermaker (1966), and Murray Wax (1971), and Margaret Mead's (1972) autobiography.

This book will draw on relatively recent examples from my (Schoepfle's) unpublished field journals. All three examples are based on observations in a school setting. They are transcriptions of (1) a full tape recording of a high school club meeting, (2) the description of an observed classroom episode recorded in a notepad, and (3) an episode based on a transcription of participant observation recalled after the event. I recorded these interactions after almost 9 months in the community.

All of these entries show that there is an inherent bias (Schoepfle, 1977). and distortion in recording observed interaction (Romney and Freeman, 1987). The first is a tendency to record interaction as a set of discrete stimulus–response incidents. That is, Person A says something, and Person B responds to what Person A said. In fact, in a group involving more than two people, many conversations may be going on at the same time and may at times intersect. The following illustrates this.

A RECORDED CLUB MEETING

[I arrived at 1600 hrs. about 10–15 minutes late. The meeting was in session, and I arrived in the middle of a dispute. Some of the girls followed me in.

The seating arrangement is such that the older girls—the sophomores, juniors, and seniors—sit on the left side of the room with the seats bunched into small groups of about four or five, while the freshman girls sit on the other side, in a block—the rows intact.]

R: [President and chairman of the meeting is standing in front of the room facing the group.] What is it going to come to,

I mean, we haven't done anything. There were three six-packs of 7-Up at the last game. That's pretty poor. [There is now an argument among the girls throughout the room. I cannot make it out from the recorder or my notes.]

RP: Quiet.

N: But what about, the thing is, there are several of us who live far off.... [Noise continues.]

RP: Shut up, CE.

TD: Have you considered the people who have to work? Who have no cars in have to walk? The lunch people live far.

R: I mean, there are a lot of people that work and who make it.

TD: But what if they can't work it out?

N: Yeah but what if...

R: But it may be we can put the scare into the people who don't work.

TD: But the same thing happened last year; and what happened? We made a rule which said that people weren't going to come in this year and there is a lot of people who did come back.... And I don't want the same thing to happen. Maybe some of you do, I don't know, but if we're going to go through with it, fine, you guys go through with it.... But the same thing's going to happen. [Pause] If there is going to be a club, they are going to come to the meetings.... There's no need to put a scare in them. What good's it going to do?

R: Well, they're going to start working.

RP: But how long?

FG: They're going to start working, but by the time you have the banquet they're going to be the same.

R: Yeah, but... That doesn't affect the working in the next few weeks.

FG: All right, but...

RP: They're going to have to pay to go to the [the basketball game].

In the next example of observed behavior, I wrote down what I saw in a steno pad. Later, I read these notes, off-site, into a sound recorder and then transcribed the recording. Both reading from the notes and transcribing from the recorder provided two opportunities for me to add anything I may have failed to recall when I was making the notes.

CLASSROOM INTERACTION FROM NOTES

[Classroom involves AL, a tall, mustachioed boy; ST, a student teacher; T, a full-time teacher; and three girls, G, G2, and G3. AL gives a speech on Israel. Nobody understands what he has driving at. The issue he says is that the Arabs threaten to cut off oil if we helped Israel. We did anyway, and they cut off the supply, so we may as well continue the original aid to Israel. He gives a figure of so many barrels a day that we may miss, and this figure purports to indicate the difficulties of continued support. The point of the class is not so much Israel as it is how to make a convincing argument on any topic.]

T: Does anybody understand it? [Some girls attempt to paraphrase. The problem is that AL is talking in terms of irony. Right.]

ST: The main difficulty is in illogical argument.

G: But this is only your opinion.

T: Did anybody consider the statistic shocking?

G: Yes.

T: Does this figure mean anything to you?

AL: A lot. [Laughter from the class]

ST: Well I think the argument is invalid.

AL: That's it?

ST: Yes. [AL sits down.]

GL: How many points are these worth?

AL: I've got another topic. [Grins and gets up to walk to the podium]

T: Sure, okay. [AL proposes a system like Jerry Lewis's March of Dimes to get money donations for a new school.]

GL: Then they would've approved the bond issue. That won't work.

ST: Besides the organization, how could you make this more familiar?

GL and G: More familiar?

ST: More personal, more forceful . . . Not "I suggest."

AL: I demand? [Laughter from the class]

ST: You've got to learn to be more forceful if you're going to convince anybody of anything.

G: [Frowns] Aaaahhhh . . . [Apparently in response to the student teacher's remarks]

T: [Looks back and forth along the rank of girls on the side with the observer's taking notes. She doesn't usually do this for such a response. This supports the observer suspicion that something here is a bit strained.]

AL: [Still at the podium. While he is there, T gives an example of a polluted stream that is now off-limits.]

G2: What if we never see a spring, like out here, in the desert? [Girls next to me say "Right on." T then gives the example of some of the local wells running dry.]

G3: How does this all tie-in?

T: Well, some of you know Mrs. OL, remember? She used to be a principal here. [Some of the class nod.] And it is out on Tucson highway. Her well ran dry. . . . I mean, give something close to home as an example. [The bell rings and immediately everybody jumps up and leaves.]

The third example is the transcription of participant observation involving me as a teacher. The discussion involved the teacher attempting to find a better means for classroom participation. After class, I wrote down the most prominent interchanges as closely as I could remember them. Then, I read these notes into a recorder and then transcribed the recording. Again, I had the chance to interject evaluations, descriptions, and any additional information for each incident I recalled. "RES" signifies the researcher; other acronyms signify individuals' codified names.

RECALLING OF CLASSROOM INTERACTION

[This transcription is an end of the day recall of interaction that the researcher, RES, had with the class. Other names are of individuals whose names have been codified.]

RI: I can't understand where you're trying to lead us.

RES: Would you prefer lectures?

(Continued)

(Continued)

Class:	No.
MC:	The material was new and we don't know what to say to it. [Several of the girls disagreed, saying that they were supposed to develop the concepts as they went along.]
RES:	[Added that this was where we were supposed to be starting with what we knew and working our way along.] Something must be wrong then.
JB:	I am for woman's lib, and I'm the only girl in the room who is. Nobody else is interested.
MP:	I disagree, I like some parts and not others.
JS:	How do you know [to JB] we aren't interested? [There is a pause.] This is the first decent start of the discussion we've had. [Laughter]
JF:	How about presenting our reports?
JB:	On our group?
RES:	I thought that might be a good idea, but I felt people would be embarrassed. [Several nods of approval from the class] Would demonstration by a panel be better?
MC:	No, we aren't in an English class. Besides, we don't have time.
KA:	You could send us out to do work on some issue and have everybody ready to talk. But it has to be controversy oh, and woman's lib is in controversy all.
RES:	Fair enough, what would be a good one? [Silence]
RC:	Also, we go from one thing to the next. One week it's monkey behavior, the next week it's kinship. [Class laughs.]
RES:	Then we should stick to something longer? [Several class members answer "Fine."] What specifically? [Silence.] What about raising children?
Class:	Yes.

In this last example, the intrusion of the observer's categories is most obvious. Nevertheless, in all three journal entries, the observations were recorded primarily in the categories of the observer (Werner & Schoepfle, 1987a). The first example is very cumbersome and difficult to use. Because every utterance is recorded, the transcription is time-consuming, and yet the duration of the interaction was only slightly more than 7 minutes. There are many unfinished sentences, interrupted thoughts, and interruptions of speech by others. These unfinished sentences invite further interpretation by the observer. On the other hand, it illustrates precisely how the participants were communicating with one another through intersecting trains of thought. (For further study on the subject of inferring trains of thought of participants, see Cicourel, 1974, and see Hamamoto, 1980, for a methodological critique.)

In the second example, the observer has clearly arranged the examples of behavior according to a progression of speakers while taking notes. Because the pen-and-notebook method of recording is slow, the observer could not record interruptions, unfinished sentences, and ramblings yet still keep up with the conversation. While the use of pen-and-paper records allow an observer to interpret some of the interaction in the setting, these categories of verbal exchanges are likely distorted.

The third example describes a recalled observed interaction between the observer and the class. Any of the biases that appeared in the second example—particularly inferences of train of thought—are even more distorted.

The potential evidentiary value of these kinds of observations, however, is acknowledged in today's legal and administrative proceedings. Ethnographers cannot address fully all of the problems and distortions of observation. However, observations—for better or worse—are the stuff of court proceedings.

THE APPLICATION OF PHOTOGRAPHY TO INTERVIEW AND OBSERVATION

Any kind of photograph can be misleading. The reason is simple: The aim of good photography is to produce a dramatic photograph, not simply an accurate depiction of events. Even the choice of a lens confers distortion.

For example, when Werner was a professional photographer, he was selected by the university Public Relations department to photograph a donor (of a substantial amount of money) and the university chancellor together. The chancellor stood over 6 feet tall, and the donor stood at only 5 feet. The assignment required that under no circumstances should the chancellor appear taller than the donor. Werner addressed this constraint by selecting a wide-angle lens. Taking advantage of its perspective, he placed the donor closer to the camera than the chancellor and was thus able to complete the assignment successfully (Werner & Schoepfle, 1987a).

Even ethnographic films are not above the suspicion of misrepresenting facts for the sake of either heightened drama or emphasis of a specific point.

Adam Marshall's film, *The Hunters*, excited every anthropologist. Nevertheless, detractors of the film's ethnographic accuracy have claimed that the Kalahari bushmen rarely, if ever, shoot giraffes because their poisoned arrows were simply inadequate to bring down so large an animal. They have claimed that the final collapse of the animal in the film was due not to the bushmen's poison arrows, but to Marshall's 30-06 rifle. (Werner & Schoepfle, 1987a, p. 283)

This case highlights the need to distinguish carefully between ethnography and history. For example, the Natsilik Eskimo films are first-rate and invaluable. However, they erred in history as well as ethnography because the film recorded the last full yearly cycle before the Natsilik were resettled into villages.

Time Continuum of Photography

One of the most valuable applications of photography in ethnography is in the photographic record as a "time machine" (Werner & Schoepfle, 1987a). From a long-term perspective, photographs taken from the same vantage point years apart can dramatically illustrate changes over the years. In addition to showing important changes, they also serve as projective techniques for consultants viewing the photos for comment. At the other time extreme, photographs taken at intervals greater than 48 frames per second have allowed ethnographers to analyze micromovements in speech among infants (Kempton, 1980) and in various kinds of dancing. As mentioned above, this kind of kinesthetic behavior is otherwise difficult to describe verbally.

Photographic information elicits different amounts and kinds of knowledge from different people. For example, photographs of a Navajo medicine man elicited volumes of valuable information about what he did on other days and in other places. On the other hand, an African American mother from south Chicago who was shown pictures of her daily activities gave minimal responses. Yet when an African American social worker used fragments of taped interviews with African

American mothers, she obtained from such "projective responses" much interesting information about the fears experienced by Black ghetto mothers in households without men. She played to them parts of an interview about male intruders, to which the reaction was dramatic: They all shared that fear and—prompted by the recorded fragments—talked about their own experiences.

With the introduction of the iPhone and digital cameras, readily available video applications can aid the ethnographer's memory by recording interactions in visual human communication too small in detail to write down. In addition, being able to show these to consultants within a short time becomes an even greater aid in fieldwork.

OBSERVATION AND EVIDENCE

So far this chapter has demonstrated the pitfalls awaiting the uninformed ethnographer and stressed the need to rely on interview to inform observations. The chapter concludes by stressing that observations must be ruthlessly examined for accuracy. Indeed, the accuracy demanded of observations should be pressed no less rigorously than for accounts from consultant interviews. Ethnographic interview and observation both need to generate facts—particularly in the increasingly litigious environments within which ethnographic findings will be applied. If the ethnographer and ethnography are to participate in a judicial process, they must be able to address the factual standards of the courts.

The ethnographer's journal requires the same precision that an ethnographer expects from the knowledge of consultants. Lubet (2018) observes that ethnography is rife with examples of studies conducted by sociologists, anthropologists, and journalists that muddle hearsay with fact. He cites studies that show how ethnographers report events communicated to them that they themselves could not verify. He cites additional examples—particularly from journalism—in which the author intentionally falsified or manufactured events to make a dramatic point or to portray it as representative of some events that the investigator themselves did not encounter. Verification thus requires writers to not only consult their own journals but also examine the credibility of published documentary sources that are sometimes used to evaluate the interviews.

To sort out how to triangulate interview information with other sources about events, all ethnographers have to take into consideration questions of *who, what, where, when, antecedent,* and *consequent*:

1. What exactly happened?
2. Who exactly was involved in this event?
3. Where did this event happen?
4. When did this event happen?
5. What were the antecedents to this event, and what were the consequents of this event?

In other words, ethnographers are eliciting facts. They often have to ask the same kind of sequence question they would ask a native consultant. They should be able to have the consultant answer questions about what happened and be able to break the answer down into its component parts. Answering questions about who was involved helps explore social networks. Such exploration may require specific names and the identification of specific individuals, at least in the fieldwork documentation.

Observation becomes more important, however, when the focus of the ethnographic fieldwork reaches beyond characterizing the knowledge and way of life of a people and evaluates the truth and factual nature of a consultant's description. There will be contradictions between Texts 1 and 2. While it may be tempting to rely on one source or record over the other, it is vitally important that the ethnographer makes every effort to *reconcile* the two.

The dramatic growth in audiovisual media for recording is too great to itemize here. Moreover, the opportunities for follow-up interviews even after leaving the field have expanded in ways unknown to previous generations of ethnographers. This fact presents both blessings and challenges, particularly in maintaining ethical relationships. Ethnographers cannot really understand a culture simply by asking people how to operate, any more than they can learn by watching alone. This interaction of observation, interview, and praxis is the fundamental property of the *participant observation* outlined in Chapter 1. Yet the transcribed interview is still the best place to start and the best means to monitor understanding of a cultural knowledge system. The interview "keeps us honest," and it does so from the beginning of research to its end.

CHAPTER 8

WRITING THE ETHNOGRAPHIC REPORT

The interviews have been planned, conducted, and analyzed. It is now time to communicate the results of the analysis to others. While the presentation of these ethnographic reports may be oral, visual, or written, they are all based on some sort of script (Spradley, 1980). As was seen earlier, the boundary between the interview and the analysis is not always sharp. Likewise, the boundary between the analysis and the report is also not sharp.

This chapter proposes four ethnographic report styles: descriptive, analytical, synthetic, and case study. The chapter begins with the descriptive style and shows how the MTQ schema, which was applied during research and analysis, can serve as a basis on which to organize the ethnographic report. The chapter also outlines how to develop the descriptive ethnography in the absence of any diagrams developed during the research. The diagrams based on the MTQ schema also aid in controlling writers' block. This is achieved partly through debriefing the researcher and partly through organizing the textual database. The chapter concludes with the authors' experience in involving the coresearchers in the report writing.

FOUR MAJOR REPORT-WRITING STYLES: DESCRIPTIVE, ANALYTICAL, SYNTHETIC, AND CASE STUDY

All ethnographies condense and organize the volumes of interview and journal data texts, photos, and other media collected during the research into a script that can be understood by someone who was not the ethnographer. The term "script" is used here to emphasize that while ethnographic reports can also include media such as photographs and motion pictures they are at some point organized into a script. The goal of writing an ethnographic report is thus to develop a script that presents the data and analysis from the field research to a wider audience.

The descriptive reporting style represents the most direct link between the cultural knowledge of the consultants that the ethnographer interviewed and observed. Centering on the MTQ schema, the ethnographer first generates the schema from the data. This generation is likely done by the end of the research itself or soon thereafter. The ethnographer then narrates these schema, preferably in front of an audience, and adds annotative remarks intended to help the audience understand how the schema works. The researcher then converts this verbal narrative to a written format. This written narrative then becomes the first draft of the written report. The procedure is simple and is a great way to start.

The analytic style breaks down information into component parts. It is a good way to present ethnographic data if the reader and audience already have some idea about the social system being described, and how it works. If they are not familiar with the culture, the analytic approach can be mystifying.

The synthetic style puts the parts together into a working whole and is the most common style of a written report. It is not, however, the most efficient way of communicating the results rapidly to relevant consumers. Writers may combine the introduction and the conclusions and put this synthetically conjoined product at the very beginning of the report. The problem with this approach is that there is no closure. This report tells the reader what they need to know up front. If they are interested, they can read more of the details and the evidence in the rest of the report. The documentation of the conclusion is contained there.

The case study uses many real-life anecdotes to illustrate the generalizations. Case studies show the functioning of the cultural and social system. The theory should not prejudice how one writes the report. There may be a theoretical point to make, but that needs to be taken into account as one begins collecting and analyzing texts. Ethnography can include many specific cases, such as eyewitness stories of events. Cases and anecdotes have an undeservedly bad reputation for being insufficient for a report. However, there is nothing to prevent the writer from collecting anecdotes in a systematic manner. To the best of our knowledge of the "classical" ethnographers, only the late Clyde Kluckhohn has ever made a generalization and then illustrated his point with a case, adding that he had collected and saved 25 additional, similar cases in a database. The synthetic description of a culture can be aided by case studies.

WHEN SCHEMA ARE NOT AVAILABLE
OR HAVE NOT BEEN GENERATED

Once the analysis is done, it may still be difficult to begin any kind of writing enterprise. One strategy that we found useful was to use debriefing. The students attending the Northwestern Ethnographic Field School found the debriefing useful, as did the Navajo coresearchers. The debriefing was useful to aid memory and as a tool to begin the writing process.

The goal of debriefing the students at the Ethnographic Field School was to assess what, and how much, they had learned. Often the students appeared at a debriefing with voluminous field notes and interview transcripts. We did not have time for a lengthy "data dump." Instead, we debriefed them for their *recollections* of what they had found. We started by asking grand-tour questions, many as simple as "Tell me what you found" or "What did you notice?" or even "What impressed you the most?" While we took notes, we also began sketching diagrams of what the students were describing. Once the students had finished reporting whatever they could recall, we would prompt them with mini-tour questions. After the students had completed the verbal debriefing, we then reiterated what we had just heard and showed the students how they might diagram what they had described. We suggested further diagrams, and we asked them to review their field notes and interview transcripts and refine or replace the diagrams that had been sketched during this debriefing. Finally, if the students did not have sufficient information on a topic, we urged them to use the last two or three weeks of their fieldwork to focus on collecting the missing information. It was here that they were informed—if they were not yet aware—that the last 90% of the research is usually conducted in the last 10% of the time.

As a culmination of their field school work, the field school directors expected all the students to present their results in front of their peers. To prepare for this presentation, the students were requested to

1. describe very briefly what they did, including where they were residing, whom they interviewed, how many interviews they

conducted; when they conducted these interviews, and any other features of the field conditions;

2. draw out, on butcher paper, the graphs or diagrams they had derived during their fieldwork (let us remember we were presenting out of doors in a wilderness setting far away from electrical outlets);

3. narrate the diagrams as clearly as possible;

4. explain briefly how their study was important to them; and

5. explain how their results might be important not only for the advancement of social science but also to help the people with whom the students had been working.

This presentation was supposed to last no longer than 10 to 15 minutes, with time at the end for questions or discussion from the field school staff and student peers. Navajo students at the Community College were enrolled at the Northwestern University Ethnographic Field School as well. The students, regardless of educational background, were expected to present a verbal report and then draft a written version of it.

Getting the Report Down on Paper: Controlling Writer's Block

Once the initial descriptive report is assembled, the problem of writer's block emerges. The paralysis one experiences when confronting the task of putting something down on paper, in fact, often arises from the panic of having *too much* to write about. An ethnographer's database is usually very rich, and it is easy to get so overwhelmed by its sheer size that one does not know where to start. The first ethnography may thus be the most difficult document to write. It might be tempting to start with the introduction. This option, however, is not always a good idea because few writers really know what they are going to write about until they finish writing it. If one is going to start with an introduction, it is best for it to assume the form of an outline. Once the report is written, the introduction may have to be rewritten—in fact, several times.

Franz Boaz, the grandfather of American anthropology, pointed out many years ago that one can start an ethnography anywhere—in any one of a culture's many patches. It does not really matter where one starts. As the writing proceeds, new insights emerge, writers discover better ways of analyzing things, forgotten questions from when the ethnographers were in the field reappear, or writers discover a more logically robust organization. It is thus best to leave the final version of the introduction to the last.

Even that observation may present a problem if the author is confronted with writer's block. Another technique to cope with this problem is to write down the ideas, in any order, then shuffle them around in various orders. This approach is also known as the "scratch list" (Werner & Schoepfle, 1987b). The steps include

1. making a list of everything that pops into one's head,

2. sorting the list of topics and subtopics, and

3. expanding these topics according to one's best judgment for the ethnographic presentations or texts.

The main point is to write down everything in telegraph style and keep adding to that list until the writer has exhausted all of their ideas. With modern word-processing software, this approach is relatively easy.

A variation of this scratch list approach is to invite a familiar colleague who will ask good questions. To keep the meeting informal and comfortable for both,

1. tell this friend what we have been doing with the ethnographic project;

2. let the friend ask questions;

3. record the proceedings, including any explanations and discussion; and

4. write out what was recorded—not verbatim (let the sound recording stimulate thoughts)—and write down any additional ideas that emerge.

After meeting with the friend, we transcribe the recorded discussion. We do not transcribe verbatim. As we listen, the digital recording stimulates our memory. We annotate or insert anything new that might appear about the ethnography that we also may wish to write about. This annotation process stimulates the memory, as it did when the ethnographer wrote his or her journals. At this point, the writers

1. use many headings and subheadings,

2. make a table of contents of the headings and subheadings,

3. reorder the titles following their best judgment for an effective presentation,

4. fill in the detailed text under the appropriate heading, and

5. write or rewrite the introduction and conclusions.

The last option is to use word frequency indexes. These can be used to start an outline, and they give an excellent indication of what is contained in the interviews. Once the keywords have been sorted, the same keywords can be repeated with the folk definitions and attributes that included them. Finally, compound folk definitions can be constructed as subtopics as well. We can actually use folk definitions exclusively and sort these into any ordered set that makes any sense to us. It is also possible to construct a list of definitions and subtopics.

ORGANIZING THE REPORT

The first step is to gather together the individual folk definitions, diagrams, and quotes. The next step is to group them into different themes. As different themes emerge, one can add quotes that enhance or clarify these themes. These notes and themes, in turn, may also be shared with the consultants. Finally, these definitions can then be grouped in a way that is meaningful to the writer. These groups do not look necessarily like a report, but they expose or highlight the topics that must be covered later in writing the report.

One variant of sorting is to give an oral report and record it along with any questions the audience may have. As in a scratch list, the steps help sort out what is important and provide a potential presentation order.

Long ago, in writing the *Six Navajo School Ethnographies* (Werner et al., 1976), the authors organized the texts from each consultant into folk definitions, or some kind of taxonomic trees or lattice structures, as discussed in the earlier chapters. We then put these on white, 5- by 8-inch cards. Then we combined the white cards dealing with the same topics on yellow cards. For example, each student classified his or her fellow classmates. That classification was entered onto the white cards. The combined classification of all students was entered onto a yellow card. The ethnographers used various notational conventions to keep track of the sources of the data, especially if there were discrepancies. Then, they had a conference. Since the project consisted of several ethnographers, they discussed the order in which their materials should be presented. After the discussion, they rearranged the yellow cards in the order agreed on and started writing.

What Constitutes an Adequate Text Database?

It is rare that an ethnographic project will reach the state of diminishing returns—when no more information seems to be found. The answer to this question thus seems dictated more by the available time than by considerations of ethnographic adequacy. Moreover, we recognize that the way data are grouped is guided by the practical and theoretical goals of the ethnography when we undertake it.

Once the writers have indexed not only the interviews but also their journal entries, they can begin writing. There are many different writing styles for ethnography, and it is important to keep in mind that the long paper or monograph is not necessarily the best way to communicate ethnographic insights. Ethnographers must always be on the lookout for other, more effective ways. Oral presentation is one approach. Once we give an oral presentation, we may be in a better position to judge people's responses. Both the field school debriefing and talking to a friend are good examples.

Bulkiness of Documents in Reports and Records: Work Papers

A readable report must indicate where to put information that is important to the analysis of the ethnography but that the reader would not want to review. Not all of the analysis will be placed in the report itself. For example, field notes and other interview texts may become part of the ethnographer's permanent record but should not be available to the public. Information also needs to be withheld out of consideration for privacy, but it should not be destroyed. It may have unanticipated value for later research. Legal issues may arise where consulting this information might become important. Finally, information obtained from research conducted for a government or corporate entity might be important to maintain for the administrative record.

Records may also need to be available for peer review, for administrative review, or in a court of law. One solution, used by government and some corporate agencies, is to store them in files of work papers. While work papers are often associated with audits, they are relevant to ethnography as well. According to the U.S. Government Accountability Office (1998),

> workpapers provide documentation on the scope of the audit and the diligence with which it was completed. Audit workpapers (1) assist in planning the audit; (2) record the procedures applied, tests performed, and evidence gathered; (3) provide support for technical conclusions; and (4) provide the basis for review by management. Audit workpapers also provide the principal support for the auditor's report, which is to be provided to the audited taxpayer, on findings and conclusions about the taxpayer's correct tax liability. (p. 2)

Among other elements, such papers contain data analysis, tentative conclusions, and recorded or transcribed interviews. They are not part of a report but are part of the administrative record, which provides the means of tracking any analysis that was done. They are thus available should further analysis or reanalysis be necessary. Ethnography, as we mentioned previously, will have more demands made on it as its practitioners are challenged for their expertise (see Chapter 7).

A FINAL WORD ON NATIVE CORESEARCHERS

No matter how simple the presentation may be, we must always remember that every ethnography makes a contribution to social theory. It may not be large or obvious, but it is a contribution. Thus, it is important to involve the coresearchers in the report writing as well as in the oral presentations. They have made valuable contributions. Presentations are part of their continued integration into the research enterprise itself. We thus strongly urge co-ethnographers to be involved in oral presentations at the same anthropological association, meetings, regional scientific associations, or conventions attended by the ethnographers.

Initial reactions by the coresearchers are not always positive. In objecting, they have asked rhetorically, "Why do we need to present papers? This is all about our lives, and we should have a right to present our lives in any way we see fit—or not to present anything about our lives at all." It may be necessary to examine the context behind these objections. For example, while many native co-ethnographers have knowledge of the research subject, they have not likely had experience with presentations in front of nonnative audiences, and these can be intimidating.

Part of the solution is to rehearse the presentations in front of one another or peers (and the ethnographer) first, as if they were actually in front of an audience. Again, the descriptive report is vital. This kind of involvement helps discourage the patronizing attitude toward the "native opinion" often presented at these meetings. Instead, the coresearchers are presenting data just like everyone else. Their contribution to the research effort is far more important than just an opinion, so we expect them to present data and analysis as well.

The descriptive study report most easily links the coresearchers to the presentation. Since the coresearchers sometimes do not have experience in expository writing, we begin by first interviewing them to see what they want to present and what information they have brought for the review. From these debriefing interviews, we present back to the coresearchers what they have presented to us. We would then recommend the same kinds of diagrams as we have presented in this volume. We work with the coresearchers to refine and improve the diagrams. These diagrams will then become the centerpiece of the presentations.

We presented papers to regional scholarly associations such as the American Association for the Advancement of Science, South West Social Sciences Association, American Anthropological Association, and Society for Applied Anthropology. The schemata of these presentations were usually drafted in both Navajo and English. Then, the presentations were verbally delivered. These presentations, in turn, also gave the co-ethnographers standing to present these same diagram-based direct studies to tribal governmental and local political organizations. The Navajo ethnographers on these projects reported acquiring standing with other Navajo community members and within the overall tribal political system.

Finally, although employment opportunities were enhanced for the Navajo ethnographers after these projects, these opportunities were not necessarily in research. This development was good because we often had to confront burnout in the research teams. After a certain point, the co-ethnographers took on jobs elsewhere within the tribal government, within education, or within the developing tribal college systems. We have thus tended to keep track of our ethnographic colleagues long after the research project was over. Many have become and remained our friends through the years.

REFERENCES

Aberle, D. F. (1987). Distinguished Lecture: What kind of science is anthropology? *American Anthropologist, 89*(3), 551–566. https://doi.org/10.1525/aa.1987.89.3.02a00010

Agar, M. H. (2006). An ethnography by any other name. *Forum: Qualitative Social Research Sozialforschung, 7*(4), Art. 36. https://www.qualitative-research.net/index.php/fqs/article/view/177/396

Agar, M. H. (2010). On the ethnographic part of the mix: A multi-genre tale of the field. *Organizational Research Methods, 13*(2), 286–303. https://doi.org/10.1177/1094428109340040

Ahern, J. (1979). *Results from the Tower Rock Community Study* [Unpublished manuscript]. Northwestern University Ethnographic Field School.

Albisetti, C., & Venturelli, A. J. (1962). *Encyclopedia Bororo* (2 vols.). Instituto de Pesquisas Etnográficas, Faculdade Dom Aquino de Filosofía, Ciências e Letras.

American Anthropological Association. (2004). *American Anthropological Association statement on ethnography and institutional review boards: Adopted by AAA Executive Board June 4, 2004.* http://research.fiu.edu/documents/irb/documents/ethnographyReview.pdf

Austin-Garrison, M. A. (2017). Step-by-step translation: *Awę́ę́ Łééchąą'í Yiltsąągo Yeełt'é* (translated from the original Navajo). In O. Werner (Ed.), *On translation: Toward a theory of translation* (pp. 11–13). Northwestern University.

Beebe, J. (2001). *Rapid assessment process: An introduction.* Alta Mira Press.

Begishe, K. Y., Schoepfle, G. M., & Platero, D. (1981). *N7ts1hakees: Navajo thought development* (First Quarterly Progress Report of the Ethnographic and Sociolinguistic Survey of Bilingual Education Programs). U.S. Office of Education.

Benedict, R. (1959). *Patterns of culture.* Houghton Mifflin.

Bidney, D. (1967). *Theoretical anthropology.* Columbia University Press. https://doi.org/10.7312/bidn94356

Blount, B., Jacob, S., Weeks, P., & Jepson, M. (2015). Testing cognitive ethnography: Mixed methods in developing indicators of well-being in fishing communities. *Human Organization, 74*(1), 1–15.

Bohannan, P. J., Powers, W. T., & Schoepfle, G. M. (1974). Systems conflict in the learning alliance. In J. L. Stiles (Ed.), *Theories for teaching* (chap. 4). Dodd, Mead.

Bolles, R. N. (2018). *What color is your parachute?* Ten Speed Press.

Briggs, J. (1970). *Never in anger: Portrait of an Eskimo family.* Harvard University Press.

Briggs, J. L. (1970). Kapluna daughter: Living with Eskimos. In P. Golde (Ed.), *Women in the field: Anthropological experiences* (pp. 19–46). Aldine. https://doi.org/10.1007/BF02805482

Britannica.com. (n.d.). Discovery. In *Encyclopedia Britannica.* https://www.britannica.com/topic/discovery-law

Bruner, J. (1990). *Acts of meaning* (Jerusalem–Harvard Lectures). Harvard University Press.

Campbell, H., Slack, J., & Diedrich, B. (2017). Mexican immigrants, anthropology, and United States law: Pragmatics, dilemmas, and ethics of expert witness testimony. *Human Organization,* 76(4), 326–334. https://doi.org/10.17730/0018-7259.76.4.326

Carome, M. A., & Department of Health & Human Services. (2003, September 22). *OHRP letter to the leaders of the Oral History Association* (Linda Shopes, Division of History, Pennsylvania Historical and Museum Commission, and Donald A. Ritchie, Senate Historical Office, United States Senate). https://www.shsu.edu/dept/office-of-research-and-sponsored-programs/documents/OHRPResponsetoOralHistories.pdf

Casagrande, J. B., & Hale, K. L. (1967). Semantic relations in Pop Ago folk definitions. In H. B. Biddle (Ed.), *Hymns with Biddle* (pp. 165–193). Mouton.

Cernea, M. (2002). *Impoverishment risks and reconstruction: A model for population displacement and resettlement.* Brookings Institution.

Chomsky, N. (1968). *Language and mind.* Harcourt Brace. https://doi.org/10.1037/e400082009-004

Cicourel, A. (1974). *Cognitive sociology: Language and meaning in social interaction.* Free Press.

Cochran, W. G. (1977). *Sampling techniques* (3rd ed.). Wiley.

Conklin, H. C. (1983). *Ethnographic atlas of Ifugao: Implications for theories of agricultural evolution in Southeast Asia.* Yale University Press.

Cooke, J. (1980, September 28). Jimmy's world. *The Washington Post.* https://www.washingtonpost.com/archive/politics/1980/09/28/jimmys-world/605f237a-7330-4a69-8433-b6da4c519120/?utm_term=.f22a8bff781b

Cited in discussion on part-whole D'Andrade, R. G. (1983). *A folk model of the mind.* Cambridge University Press.

Daubert v. Merrill Dow Pharmaceuticals, Inc., 509 U.S. 579, 113 S. Ct. 2786 (1993). https://supreme.justia.com/cases/federal/us/509/579/

DeWalt, K. M., & DeWalt, B. R. (with Weyland, C. B.). (1998). Participant observation. In R. H. Bernard (Ed.), *Handbook of methods in cultural anthropology* (pp. 259–300). Alta Mira Press.

Fanale, R. (1982). *Navajo land and land management: A century of change* [Unpublished doctoral dissertation]. Department of Anthropology, Catholic University.

Franciscan Fathers. (2015). *An ethnologic dictionary of the Navaho language.* Saint Michaels.

Fraser, B. (2009). Topic orientation markers. *Journal of Pragmatics, 41*(5), 892–898. https://doi.org/10.1016/j.pragma.2008.08.006

Freedom of Information Act, 5 U.S.C. §551–552 (1967). https://www.foia.gov/5 U.S.C.

Frye v. United States, 293 F. 1013 (D.C. Cir 1923). https://www.law.ufl.edu/_pdf/faculty/little/topic8.pdf

Garrison, E. R., & Schoepfle, G. M. (1977). *Attitudes of Navajo students toward teachers and school activities* [Paper presentation]. Joint meeting of the Society for Applied Anthropology and the Southwest Anthropological Association, San Diego, CA, United States.

Gladwin, C. H. (1989). *Ethnographic decision tree modeling* (Qualitative Research Methods Series, Vol. 19). Sage. https://doi.org/10.4135/9781412984102

Hall, E. T. (1969). *The hidden dimension.* Doubleday/Anchor.

Hamamoto, M. (1980). *Ethnoscience in the study of human interpretation* [Unpublished manuscript]. Department of Anthropology, Northwestern University.

Harwood, F. (1976). Myth, memory, and the oral tradition: Cicero in the Trobriands, *American Anthropologist, 78*(4), 783–796. https://doi.org/10.1525/aa.1976.78.4.02a00040

Herlihy, P. H. (2003a). Participatory research mapping of indigenous lands in Darien, Panama. *Human Organization, 62*(4), 315–331. https://doi.org/10.17730/humo.62.4.fu05tgkbvn2yvk8p

Herlihy, P. H., & Knapp, G. (2003b). Maps of, by, and for the peoples of Latin America. *Human Organization, 62*(4), 303–314. https://doi.org/10.17730/humo.62.4.8763apjq8u053p03

Hewitt, B. G. (1987). *The typology of subordination in Georgian and Abkhaz.* De Gruyter Mouton. https://doi.org/10.1515/9783110846768

Heyman, J. (2004). The anthropology of power-wielding bureaucracies. *Human Organization, 63*(4), 487–500. https://doi.org/10.17730/humo.63.4.m9phulu49a1l2dep

Hirsch, A. (2014). *Going to the source: The "new" Reid method and false confessions.* https://pdfs.semanticscholar.org/9f3f/d52ecc20cb9c988818403d66664278e97352.pdf

Ho, K. (2009). *Liquidated: An ethnography of Wall Street*. Duke University Press. https://doi.org/10.1515/9780822391371

Inbau, F. E., Reid, J. E., Buckley, J. P., & Jayne, B. C. (2015). *Essentials of the Reid technique: Criminal interrogation and confessions* (2nd ed.). Jones & Bartlett Learning.

Jaffrey, M. (1975). *An invitation to Indian cooking*. Random House.

Jones, P., Drury, R., & McBeath, J. (2011). Using GPS-enabled mobile computing to augment qualitative interviewing: Two case studies. *Field Methods, 23*(2), 173–187. https://doi.org/10.1177/1525822X10388467

Kempton, W. (1980). The rhythmic basis of inner actual micro-synchrony. In M. R. Key (Ed.), *The relationship of verbal and nonverbal communication* (pp. 67–76). De Gruyter Mouton. https://doi.org/10.1515/9783110813098

Kilcullen, D. (2010). *Counterinsurgency*. Cambridge University Press.

Kilcullen, D. (2013). *Out of the mountains: The coming-of-age of the urban guerrilla*. Oxford University Press.

Kluckhohn, C., & Murray, H. A. (1953). *Personality in nature, society, and culture* (2nd ed.). Knopf.

Krakauer, J. (1996). *Into the wild*. Anchor Books.

Krakauer, J. (1999). *Into thin air: A personal account of the Mount Everest disaster*. Anchor Books; Doubleday.

Krakauer, J. (2003). *Under the banner of heaven: A story of violent faith*. Anchor Books.

Lang, H., Challenor, P., & Kilworth, D. (2004). A new addition to the family of space sampling methods. *Field Methods, 16*(1), 55–69. https://doi.org/10.1177/1525822X03259281

Lazarfeld, P. F. (1967). Concept formation and measurement in the behavioral sciences: Some historical observations. In G. J. Direnzo (Ed.), *Concepts, theory, and explanation in the behavioral sciences* (pp. 144–202). Random House.

Litowitz, B., & Novy, F. (1984). Expression of the part–whole semantic relation by three- to twelve-year-old children. *Journal of Child Language, 11*(1), 159–181. https://doi.org/10.1017/S030500090000564X

Loftus, E. F. (1979). *Eyewitness testimony*. Harvard University Press.

Lubet, S. (2018). *Interrogating ethnography: Why evidence matters*. Oxford University Press.

Luria, A. R. (1969). *The mind of a mnemonist: A little book about a vast memory*. Basic Books.

Malinowski, B. (1922). *Argonauts of the Western Pacific: An account of native enterprise and adventure in the archipelago of Melanesian New Guinea*. Dutton.

Malinowsky, B. (1967). *A diary in the strictest sense of the term.* Harcourt, Brace & World.

McCarty, C. (1994). Determining sample size for surveys. *Cultural Anthropology Methods, 6*(3), 5. https://doi.org/10.1177/1525822X9400600302

Mead, M. (1966). *Writings of Ruth Benedict: An anthropologist at work.* Atherton Press.

Mead, M. (1972). *Blackberry wine: My earlier years.* Morrow.

Nader, L. (1969). Up the anthropologist: Perspectives gained from studying up. In D. Hymes (Ed.), *Reinventing anthropology* (pp. 284–311). Vintage Books.

Naroll, R. (1962). *Data quality control: A new research technique.* Free Press.

National Court Rules Committee. (2021). *Federal rules of evidence.* https://www.rulesofevidence.org/

National Park Service. (2004). *Policies for managing cultural resources.* U.S. Department of the Interior.

Offen, K. H. (2003). Narrating place and identity, or mapping Miskitu land claims in northeastern Nicaragua. *Human Organization, 62*(4), 382–392. https://doi.org/10.17730/humo.62.4.f9xgq4cu3ff88he0

O'Reilly, K. (2009). Going "native." In *Key concepts in ethnography.* Sage. https://doi.org/10.4135/9781446268308

Orlando, J. (2014). *Interrogation techniques* (OLR Research Report). https://www.cga.ct.gov/2014/rpt/2014-R-0071.htm

Palinkas, L. A., Horwitz, S. M., Green, C. A., Wisdom, J. P., Duan, N., & Hoagwood, K. (2013). Purposeful sampling for qualitative data collection and analysis in mixed method implementation research. *Administration and Policy in Mental Health and Mental Health Services Research, 42*(5), 533–544. https://doi.org/10.1007/s10488-013-0528-y

Pike, K. L. (Ed.). (1967). *Language in relation to a unified theory of structure of human behavior* (2nd ed.). De Gruyter Mouton. https://doi.org/10.1037/14786-000

Platero, D., Begishe, K. Y., & Schoepfle, G. M. (1983). *Ethnographic and sociolinguistic study of an exemplary bilingual education program: Rock Point Community School.* National Institute of Education, Diné Bi'Olta Research Associates.

Polanyi, M. (1966). *The tacit dimension.* Anchor.

Powdermaker, H. (1966). *Stranger and friend: The ways of the anthropologist.* W. W. Norton.

Quine, W. V. O. (1941). *Elementary logic.* Harvard University Press.

Redfield, R. (1930). *Tepoztalan, a Mexican village: A study of folk life.* University of Chicago Press.

Roberts, J. M. (1956). Zuni daily activities. *University of Nebraska Laboratory of Anthropology Monographs, Note Book 3*(i), 1–23.

Rodriguez, L. (2014). A cultural anthropologist as expert witness: A lesson in asking and answering the right questions. *Practicing Anthropology, 36*(3), 6–10. https://doi.org/10.17730/praa.36.3.f426250289t72072

Rohner, R. P. (Ed.). (1969). *The ethnography of Franz Boaz.* University of Chicago Press.

Romney, A. K., & Freeman, S. C. (1987). Cognitive structure and informant accuracy. *American Anthropologist, 89*(2), 310–325. https://doi.org/10.1525/aa.1987.89.2.02a00020

Romney, A. K, Weller, S. C., & Batchelder, W. H. (1986). Culture as consensus: A theory of culture and informant accuracy. *American Anthropologist, 88*(2), 313–338. https://doi.org/10.1525/aa.1986.88.2.02a00020

Rosen, L. (1977). The anthropologist as expert witness. *American Anthropologist, 79*(3), 555–578. https://doi.org/10.1525/aa.1977.79.3.02a00020

Ryan, G. W., & Bernard, H. R. (2006). Testing and ethnographic decision tree model on a national sample: Recycling beverage cans. *Human Organization, 65*(1), 103–114. https://doi.org/10.17730/humo.65.1.884p8d1a2hxxnk79

Ryle, G. (1946). *Knowing how and knowing that: Proceedings of the Aristotelian Society.* Harrison.

Sanjek, R. (1991). The ethnographic present. *Man, 26*(4), 609–628. https://doi.org/10.2307/2803772

Schoepfle, G. M. (1977). *Nogales High School: Peer group and institution in a Mexican–American border town* [Unpublished doctoral dissertation]. Department of Anthropology, Northwestern University.

Schoepfle, G. M., Begishe, K. Y., Morgan, R. T., John, J., Thomas, H., & Tso, B. (1979, May 25). *A study of Navajo perceptions of the impact of environmental changes relating to energy resources development* (ED 197916, Contract No. 68-01-3868). U.S. Environmental Protection Agency.

Schoepfle, M., Burton, M., & Begishe, K. (1984). Navajo attitudes toward development and change: A unified ethnographic and survey approach to an understanding of their future. *American Anthropologist, 86*(4), 885–904. https://doi.org/10.1525/aa.1984.86.4.02a00040

Schoepfle, M., Burton, M., & Morgan, F. (1984). Navajos and energy development: Economic decision making under political uncertainty. *Human Organization, 43*(3), 265–276. https://doi.org/10.17730/humo.43.3.d682555726827052

Schoepfle, G. M., Nabahe, K., Johnson, A., & Upshaw, L. (1982). *Final report: Navajo pastoral land use and conservation in modern ecological and economic contexts* (NSF/ISP-82015). National Science Foundation; Navajo Community College.

Schoepfle, G. M., Topper, M. D., & Fisher, L. E. (1974). Operational analysis of culture and the operation of ethnography: A re-conciliation. *Culture and Cognition, 7*, 379–406.

Schoepfle, G. M., & Werner, O. (1999). Ethnographic debriefing. *Field Methods, 11*(2), 158–165. https://doi.org/10.1177/1525822X9901100206

Scudder, T. (1973). Summary: Resettlement. In W. C. Ackermann, G. F. White, & E. B. Worthington (Eds.), *Man-made lakes: Their problems and environmental effects* (Geophysical Monograph Series No. 17). American Geophysical Union.

Scudder, T. (1979). *Expected impacts of compulsory relocation on Navajos, with special emphasis on relocation from the former Joint Use Area, required by PL 93 531.* Institute for Development Anthropology Inc.

Senft, G. (1997). Bronislaw Kasper Malinowski. In *Handbook of pragmatics online* (pp. 1–16). John Benjamin.

Shweder, R. A., & D'Andrade, R. G. (1980). The systematic distortion hypothesis. In R. A. Schweder (Ed.), *Fallible judgement in behavioral research* (pp. 37–58; New Directions for Methodology of Social and Behavioral Science, Vol. 4). Jossey-Bass.

Sieber, J. E., & Tolich, M. B. (2013). *Ethically responsible research.* Sage. https://doi .org/10.4135/9781506335162

Spradley, J. P. (1970). *You owe yourself a drunk: An ethnography of urban nomads.* Little, Brown.

Spradley, J. P. (1974, June). Consultation on the conduct of ethnography at the Navajo Division of Education, Window Rock, AZ, United States.

Spradley, J. P. (1980). *Participant observation.* Holt Rinehart & Winston.

Tonigan, R. F. (1982). *The Kirtland Petition Study, Central Consolidated School District, New Mexico.* Richard F. Tonigan Associates.

Topper, M. D. (1972). *The daily life of a traditional Navajo household, and ethnographic study of human daily activities* [Unpublished doctoral dissertation]. Department of Anthropology, Northwestern University.

Topper, M. D., Nations, J. D., Detweiler, R., & Stovall, J. A. (1974). *The ethnography of a day: Some new developments* [Unpublished manuscript]. Department of Anthropology, Northwestern University.

Topper, M. L. (1976). The cultural approach, verbal action plans, and alcohol research. In M. W. Everett, J. O. Waddell, & D. B. Heath (Eds.), *Cross-cultural approaches to the study of alcohol: An interdisciplinary perspective* (pp. 379–402). De Gruyter Mouton.

Topper, M. L. (1980). Drinking as an expression of status: Navajo male adolescents. In J. O. Waddell & M. W. Everett (Eds.), *Drinking behavior among southwestern Indians: An anthropological perspective* (pp. 103–147). University of Arizona Press.

U.S. Code of Federal Regulations. (n.d.). Office of the Federal Register. https://www .govinfo.gov/app/collection/cfr

U.S. General Accounting Office. (1994). *Pollution prevention: EPA should re-examine the objectives and sustainability of state programs* (Report to the Chairman, Subcommittee on Environment, Energy, and Natural Resources, Committee on Government Operations, House of Representatives, GAO/PE MD-94-8).

U.S. Government Accountability Office. (1998). *IRS audits: Workpapers lack documentation of supervisory review* (Report to the Chairman, Subcommittee on Oversight, Committee on Ways and Means, House of Representatives, GAO/GGD-98-98). https://www.gao.gov/products/GGD-98-98

U.S. Office of Management and Budget. (2002, February 22). Guidelines for ensuring and maximizing the quality, objectivity, utility, and integrity of information disseminated by federal agencies. *Federal Register.* https://www.federalregister.gov/ documents/2002/02/22/R2-59/guidelines-for-ensuring-and-maximizing-the-quality-objectivity-utility-and-integrity-of-information

Wagner, R. (1975). *The invention of culture.* University of Chicago Press.

Wax, M. (1971). *Doing fieldwork: Warnings and advice.* University of Chicago Press.

Werner, O. (1989). Short takes: Keeping track of your interviews I. *Field Methods, 1*(1), 6–7. https://doi.org/10.1177%2F1525822X8900100105

Werner, O. (1993). *Culture through language* [Unpublished master's thesis]. Northwestern University.

Werner, O. (1999). When recording is impossible. *Field Methods, 11*(1), 71–76. https:// doi.org/10.1177/1525822X9901100108

Werner, O., Austin, M., & Begishe, K. Y. (1976). *Navajo ethnomedical encyclopedia* (American Indian/Alaska Native Health Research Advisory Council Report Fiscal Year 2010). U.S. Office of Management and Budget.

Werner, O., Begishe, K. Y., Austin-Garrison, M. A., & Werner, J. (1986). *The anatomical atlas of the Navajo.* Native American Materials Development Center.

Werner, O., & Bernard, H. R. (1994). Short Take 13: Ethnographic sampling. *Cultural Anthropology Methods, 6*(2), 7–9. https://doi.org/10.1177/1525822X9400600203

Werner, O., & Schoepfle, G. M. (1987a). *Systematic fieldwork: Vol. 1. Foundations of ethnography and interviewing.* Sage.

Werner, O., & Schoepfle, G. M. (1987b). *Systematic fieldwork: Vol. 2. Ethnographic analysis and data management.* Sage.

Werner, O., & Schoepfle, G. M. (1993). *Culture through language: Doing systematic field work: A how to do book on ethnographies* [Unpublished manuscript, Philosophy B-10]. Northwestern University.

Werner, O., Schoepfle, G. M., Bouck, D., Roan, L., & Yazzie, K. (1976). *Six Navajo school ethnographies*. Navajo Division of Education.

Werner, O., & Topper, M. D. (1976). On the theoretical unity of ethnoscience lexicography and cognitive ethnography. In C. Ramsch (Ed.), *Semantics: Theory and application* (pp. 111–144). Proceedings of the Georgetown University Round Table on Languages and Linguistics. Georgetown University Press.

White, D. R., Burton, M. L., & Brudner, L. A. (1977). Entailment theory and method: A cross-cultural analysis of the sexual division of labor. *Behavioral Science Research, 12*(1), 1–24. https://doi.org/10.1177/106939717701200101

White, D. R., & McCann, H. G. (1981). *Material and probabilistic entailment analysis: Multivariate analysis of "if . . . then" statements* [Unpublished master's thesis]. School of Social Sciences, University of California–Irvine.

Whiting, A. J., & Whiting, B. (1970). Methods for observing and recording behavior. In R. Naroll & R. Cohen (Eds.), *A handbook of method in cultural anthropology* (pp. 283–315). Columbia University Press.

Wladyka, D., & Yaworski, W. (2017). The impact of researchers' perceptions of insecurity and organized crime on fieldwork in Central America and Mexico. *Human Organization, 76*(4), 370–379. https://doi.org/10.17730/0018-7259.76.4.370

INDEX